# SAQs for the Final FRCA

# SAQs for the Final FRCA

**Dr James Nickells FRCA**
**Dr Andy Georgiou FRCA**
**Dr Ben Walton FRCA**
North Bristol NHS Trust
Bristol

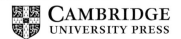

CAMBRIDGE UNIVERSITY PRESS
Cambridge, New York, Melbourne, Madrid, Cape Town, Singapore, São Paulo, Delhi

Cambridge University Press
The Edinburgh Building, Cambridge CB2 8RU, UK

Published in the United States of America by Cambridge University Press, New York

www.cambridge.org
Information on this title: www.cambridge.org/9780521739030

First published 2009

Printed in the United Kingdom at the University Press, Cambridge

*A catalogue record for this publication is available from the British Library*

ISBN 978-0-521-73903-0 paperback

Every effort has been made in preparing this publication to provide accurate and up-to-date
information which is in accord with accepted standards and practice at the time of
publication. Although case histories are drawn from actual cases, every effort has been
made to disguise the identities of the individuals involved. Nevertheless, the authors,
editors and publishers can make no warranties that the information contained herein is
totally free from error, not least because clinical standards are constantly changing through
research and regulation. The authors, editors and publishers therefore disclaim all liability
for direct or consequential damages resulting from the use of material contained in this
publication. Readers are strongly advised to pay careful attention to information provided
by the manufacturer of any drugs or equipment that they plan to use.

*From James*
*To the memory of Tessa Whitton, who was always fabulous and continues to be an inspiration.*

*From Andy*
*To my parents, Maria and Sotos, without whom I wouldn't have got this far, and to Lindsay, whose support for this exam was unfailing.*

*From Ben*
*To Joseph and Isabella.*

# Contents

Contents

# Acknowledgements

Thank you to Drs Will English, Mark Porter, James Sidney and Sara-Catrin Cook for their help in the preparation of this manuscript.

Thank you also to all the delegates who have attended and provided feedback on The Frenchay Final FRCA Crammer Course. What we learnt from you has been invaluable in devising and writing these papers.

# Introduction

'Know your enemy,
know yourself,
and your victory will not be threatened.
Know the weather,
know the terrain,
and your victory will be complete.'

Sun Tzu's Art of War, 496 BC

So, if you are reading this we guess the exam is on the horizon and you are looking for some help with the dreaded Final FRCA Short Answer Question (SAQ) paper. Well fear not, as with a little preparation and the right level of knowledge, the SAQ paper is in many ways the easiest part of the Final Examination to pass. 'They would say that' you may say to yourself but it is true. The SAQ paper rarely throws up any true 'curve balls' as, when setting the paper, the examiners have to identify topics that are important, evidence-based and represent widespread contemporary practice. This means that you are unlikely to have to deal with a historical subject such as althesin, a controversial subject such as steroids in sepsis or a subject that is not in widespread practice such as xenon (this may be fair game in the MCQ). You can even fail a substantial number of questions and still achieve a pass. As Sun Tzu said above, for your victory not to be threatened you must first know your enemy. To let you truly understand your enemy, we would like to deal with some frequently asked questions about the SAQ paper.

James Nickells<br>Andy Georgiou<br>Ben Walton

# SAQ FAQs

## The Final FRCA: what is the point?

The Royal College of Anaesthetists (the College) has a number of duties when it is examining anaesthetists for Final FRCA. It has to

– assess whether you will have enough knowledge to handle life as a consultant. In education-speak, this means that the exam is criterion-referenced. It is designed to assess what you can do rather than where you sit within the exam-sitting cohort. This should mean that in theory, everyone could pass any given sitting of the Final FRCA. Now there's a happy thought (although equally, everyone could fail!).

– assess whether you can appreciate both sides of an argument. The College likes candidates, by the time they sit the Final FRCA, to be able to grasp concepts and principles about anaesthesia. In addition to the knowledge base you amassed for the Primary Examination, you should have a good grasp of the current literature and an opinion on areas of controversy.

– show that the College is doing the right thing. Hence the focus on safety, and up-to-date, topical, scientific, widely accepted subjects.

## What does the SAQ paper consist of?

You have to write 12 questions in 3 hours. That is 15 minutes per question, maximum. You currently have six booklets (Blue, Pink, Green, and Yellow, Orange and White).

The questions are printed in the booklets with one at the front and one halfway through.

## When is the paper set?

Preliminary work will have been under way since the previous written paper. The paper is finalised about 6 weeks before the written exam.

## Should I answer the questions in order?

We would recommend that you do answer the questions in order. Some people like to answer questions they find easy first of all in the hope that inspiration will have struck when the difficult questions are tackled. This means that not only do they make life difficult for themselves fumbling between all the different coloured booklets, but that they are also going to end up tackling the most difficult questions when they are most tired and time pressure is at its worst.

## How is my mark calculated?

In the exam, questions are marked out of 20. Of those, 2 marks are given for clarity, judgement and the ability to prioritise. In a recent personal communication with an examiner, we were told

> We are looking for safe, sensible, answers that avoid a 'scatter gun' approach that includes anything that may (or may not) be distantly relevant. Such an answer will not gain the marks for judgement and the ability to prioritise. …If a candidate makes a serious or dangerous error … more than 2 marks may be withheld. A clear reason must be recorded for this.

The remaining 18 marks are scored comparing inclusions in your answer with points on a model answer plan. He went on to say

> The Examiners at Paper Setting Day and Standard Setting Day agree what marks can be given for each section and have in their marking proforma aspects of the answer which can be considered 'Essential', 'Desirable' and 'Supplementary' although it is NOT a tick-box scheme.
>
> The scores for each of the 12 questions are added and compared to the total pass mark set by the Examiners. However, the actual pass mark is moved downwards statistically because we know the SAQ currently has a reliability of 73% (*reliability means the ability of an exam to yield similar evaluations of a candidate's ability over repeated administrations with some degree of statistical certainty*). The 2+ marks are derived statistically.

The exact number passing is unpredictable for any given paper as the pass mark is shifted to represent the quality of that exam's cohort. You may fail the majority of the

Table 1. *Distribution of question by sub-specialty*

| | Total number of questions in 10 papers | % per paper | Average per paper |
|---|---|---|---|
| General anaesthesia | 41 | 34.2 | 4.1 |
| Intensive care | 24 | 20 | 2.4 |
| Paediatrics | 13 | 10.8 | 1.3 |
| Physiology, physics and equipment | 10 | 8.3 | 1.0 |
| Pharmacology | 9 | 7.5 | 0.9 |
| Anatomy | 8 | 6.7 | 0.8 |
| Obstetrics | 8 | 6.7 | 0.8 |
| Acute and chronic pain | 7 | 5.8 | 0.7 |

questions and still proceed to the oral exam stage, provided you pass the MCQ paper. Prior to 2007 the approximate standard to achieve an overall '2' on the SAQ paper was usually to score a minimum of around six '1+' and six '2'. It is thought that the modern scheme would be likely to equate to a similar standard.

You must answer all the questions. Any question that appears unattempted will score 0 and will lead to a 1 for the paper and automatic removal from the exam. Leaving a question unanswered is as good as not bothering to turn up on the day. Answer all the questions.

The College has stated that from September 2009 the MCQ and Short Answer Questions (SAQ) examination marks will be added together to give a single result. Both papers will carry equal weight. The pass marks for each part of the examination will be calculated in the current way. The pass mark for the combined examination will be the sum of the pass marks of the two papers. The written examination will stand apart from the viva examination, it will be pass/fail and must be passed before applying to sit the vivas. A pass in the written examination will be valid for two years.

## How are the sub-specialties represented in the paper?

In the previous 10 papers we found the distribution shown in Table 1. This pattern has not changed much since the first paper in 1996. You will have to face about four general anaesthesia questions, two intensive care questions and about one each of the other disciplines. If, for example, you find anatomy really difficult and decided to leave it out of your revision plan, you would have to sit three papers to hit one that had no anatomy question. The advice for revision is therefore that you do have to spread your revision time across all the subject areas.

## Are questions repeated?

When the SAQ paper was originally developed in 1996, there was a habit of regularly repeating questions from previous exams. This stopped after a few years but has started to re-occur. In the April 2008 paper, two of the 12 questions were repeated from a recent paper. The perceived view is that the College may repeat questions which were thought to be strong, but were answered poorly. This raises the question 'Is it worthwhile going through past papers?' Regardless of whether the College is repeating SAQs, we would maintain that it is definitely worth going through the past SAQs and at least formulating answer plans and checking that your knowledge covers the questions. This returns to the idea that the questions are relevant, contemporary and testing widespread, non-controversial, evidence-based topic areas. In total they cover a substantial part of the Final FRCA syllabus and knowledge gained may help with the SAQ and will certainly help with the MCQ.

## How should I prepare?

We talk later in this section under 'How should I use this book' about some aspects of preparation such as choosing the right pen. Other simple tactics may also prevent you self-destructing. Do whatever you can beforehand to minimise your stress on the day. Pack your bag the night before and go to bed early. Try to avoid an unreliable 3-hour train journey on the morning of the exam. If possible, stay overnight as close to the exam room as possible (within reason – no camping on the steps). Get a good breakfast and something to drink. If like most anaesthetists you have a coffee habit, get some on board. A caffeine slump 2 hours in will not help you. Having to leave the SAQ paper for an urgent bathroom visit is a recipe for disaster. This will take at least 10 minutes, which will seriously disrupt your timing. Deal with this before you walk into the exam room. Depending on your position on the healthy scale, nicotine patches or dried fruit may help you get through the morning. One is taken orally and the other transdermally. Don't get them the wrong way round.

## What is the best answer plan tactic?

There are a number of answer plan tactics that different people swear by.

Some people are able to sit down and write for 15 minutes in an ordered way without an answer plan. In general this is difficult to do without missing or under-representing some area of the question. You also do not allow yourself any time to order your thoughts. If you can write essays purely using an answer plan held in your brain without losing content, then this is the most time-efficient tactic. Most mere mortals will not be able to use this tactic effectively. Some sort of written answer plan will therefore be required.

Substantial, structured answer plans are at the other end of the spectrum and are to be discouraged. They will use up too much of your precious 15 minutes per question that should be used for writing down content.

Some course organisers for The Final SAQ paper advocate spending the first hour writing all 12 of your answer plans before writing any of your essays. The theory is that this will allow your subconscious to work on all the questions and pull out all deeply held knowledge. I am unaware of this tactic having been shown to be more effective and it would seem to us to be counterintuitive, as a significant amount of time would be lost writing answer plans that should be used for writing content down on the page.

Other people like to jot down 10 or so words and phrases at the top of their answer to remind themselves of a structure or of areas that they are concerned they may miss out. This does work for some people.

We recommend a slightly different tactic that seems to be effective for most people. This is a rolling plan that develops into your final answer. For example in the question 'Describe the drugs used in the management of pre-eclampsia', the different drugs or drug groups would initially be written in the booklet with half a side gap between each one. Once you are happy you have remembered most of the major drugs, you then go back and pad out each section with good content. Remember to leave more space for the main areas of the answer. It is best to leave too big a gap rather than too small. An answer with gaps between paragraphs looks acceptable, whereas a cramped up answer with arrows re-directing the reader to addendum sections looks poor. Learn how much you write for a full 15-minute essay and how much for each 10% of that time. This will also allow you to keep to time. The unique value of this tactic is that everything you put down in your answer plan gets incorporated into your final answer.

The most important factor with an answer plan tactic is that you have decided on one prior to the exam, tried it out on a number of occasions and found it to work well for you.

## How should I start an answer?

When starting an answer, it is an excellent idea to start with what we call 'The phrase that pays'. This is a succinct sentence that immediately demonstrates to the examiner that you know what you are talking about. (This is also a handy habit to get into for the vivas.) The phrase that pays will need to be crafted for each individual question. It may just be a perfect definition, or a description of a classification system. It may be the initial set-up for performing a block. Whatever form it takes for any given question, it will immediately comfort the examiner that you are knowledgeable and well organised.

## What do the stems mean?

The stem of the question is the initial section and indicates to the candidate the style and depth in which the examiners wish the question to be answered. Some of the stems are self-evident, such as 'List...' or 'Draw...'. Some are slightly more subtle in their meaning. In 1996 the essay part of the Final FRCA was reduced from five out of seven 30-minute essays to twelve 15-minute compulsory SAQs. The new paper saw the paper's stems rapidly change. Gone were the 'Compare and contrast, Criticise, Evaluate, Interpret, Justify, Relate, Review' and 'Trace'. In came 'List, What is.., Define, Discuss, How can..., What do you understand by the term..., Classify...'. As the exam has evolved, with more multi-part questions, emphatic stems that require discrete answers have become widespread. The College still requires some evidence that the candidate can assimilate information and process principles and concepts. The examiners do therefore also use some descriptive stems. These usually call for a more succinct paragraph than the descriptive stems of the old exam, and include 'Write brief notes on..., Outline..., Summarise..., Describe..., Explain..., Discuss...'.

'Write a guideline...' has come up in the past (April 2002), but is a rare beastie. It has probably proven to be unpopular as we are all aware that it takes committees many months to agree on even simple guidelines. Using a box diagram may be a way to tackle such a question. If you do need to draw a flow or box diagram, write all the text you are planning in first before drawing the boundaries around all the boxes and connecting the arrows

'Draw...' tends to polarise the candidates for the exam into two distinct groups. The first see this as an absolute breeze and the opportunity for easy marks. The second group feels their hearts sink and regress back to performing badly at GCSE Art. This is not a drawing competition but draw does mean draw. When revising learn how to draw simple reproducible line diagrams. There are a number of tips that help most people improve their performance on a 'draw' question.

Make sure your drawing has a title. This may get you a point on its own.
If you are asked to draw the anatomical relations to a specific structure, such as median nerve at the wrist in cross section, draw that object in first, then the anatomical relations and finally put the skin boundary in. Do not start by drawing the oval skin boundary in first and then trying to cram all the anatomy within that boundary.
If you are asked to draw an anatomical space (e.g. femoral triangle), it is usually best to start with a large drawing of the boundaries. Be guided by the question.
Draw BIG. Use the whole page.
Neatly label everything.
Do not be limited to nerves, arteries and veins. There may well be some marks available for labelling 'loose connective tissue' or 'lymph nodes'.

Use the time available. Drawing questions are often particularly poorly timed by candidates, who either take a few seconds and move on, missing lots of easy extra marks, or draw something beautiful but overly time-consuming.

'Write a letter to a GP…' has come up before but is also pretty rare. For this answer, notes won't do. The letter does not, however, need to be elaborate and could be as simple as:

'Dear Sir/Madam,
Thank you for asking me to review this gentleman with a strong family history of malignant hyperpyrexia. Advice regarding future anaesthetics would include….'

You will need to write in sentences and finish it off in a formal fashion. You should not sign or write your name.

## What about keywords?

When initially reading a question it is often easy to identify keywords that allow you to determine what the examiner is trying to ask and focus in on the precise nature of the question. This will unlock the main points of the question and stop you missing the point. For example in the question:

'You are asked to see a 2-year-old boy in the Emergency Department who has stridor and a barking cough. He is febrile and is sitting upright with suprasternal and subcostal recessions. What is stridor and what does it indicate? List the possible causes of stridor in a child of this age, indicating which is the most likely in this case. Outline your initial management of this child in the Emergency Department. *Oct 2007*'. Underlining the keywords would give:

'You are asked to see a 2-year-old boy in the Emergency Department who has stridor and a barking cough. He is febrile and is sitting upright with suprasternal and subcostal recessions. What is stridor and what does it indicate? List the possible causes of stridor in a child of this age, indicating which is the most likely in this case. Outline your initial management of this child in the Emergency Department.' By highlighting keywords, when attempting the last part of the question you would focus your answer only on initial management, only on a child with this clinical picture and only in the Emergency Department. This may stop you wasting valuable time discussing irrelevant aspects of management.

## How should I strike a balance between detailed and comprehensive answers?

Usually the key is the stem of the question. Consider the following four variations on a question about factors that reduce MAC:

List the factors that reduce MAC
Discuss factors that reduce MAC.
State three factors that may reduce MAC and outline why
What is the single most important factor that may reduce MAC? Why?

If you were to list all the physiological, pathological and pharmacological factors that reduce MAC, you would have a very long list. Equally, a detailed description of age and MAC would also easily fill a 15-minute essay. In the questions here, the earlier ones call for a broad comprehensive list and the latter questions are asking for more detail on individual factors on the list

## How do I avoid missing detail?

Detail in a question is often the subtle stuff that lifts your answer from being a fail to a pass or a pass to a good pass. As with keywords, the main advice for catching detail is the same. Read the question. Once you have captured all the major content, think broadly around the definitions of all the keywords. For example, if you are asked a question on the drugs used in the management of pre-eclampsia, your major content will be down the line of the classic anti-hypertensive agents and magnesium. If you then look back at the question and think to yourself 'What other drugs do I regularly give patients with pre-eclampsia?' it won't be too long before you come up with the answer that you insert an epidural and give bupivacaine. This gives you a whole new avenue to explore and will score you extra marks.

## Should I use references?

Most people are aware of a colleague who is a walking version of PubMed; able to drop perfect references in to back up all conversations about controversial topics. Most of us do not work this way and the choice of whether or not to add relevant references into an SAQ may cause anxiety. This also has relevance for revision. Should you be memorising all those references or using your time and brain units for something else? Let us consider an example:

For the question 'What is the ideal haemoglobin level for a patient on the critical care unit?' the following options are available when attempting your 'Phrase that pays':

– Studies have shown that a haemoglobin of 7g/dl is associated with improved outcome.
– In April 1999, The Canadian Clinical Trials Group showed that a haemoglobin of 7g/dl is associated with improved outcome.
– Studies have shown that a haemoglobin of 7g/dl is associated with improved outcome. (Multicenter, Randomised, Controlled Clinical Trial of Transfusion Requirements in Critical Care Canadian Critical Care Trials Group, *E Bi Gum*; 341:309–317, Feb 11, 1999.)

The third option is not only the work of madness, it is also incorrect. Attempting to put anything like full references into an SAQ is to be discouraged. The first and second options are both acceptable, and would probably score you similar points. The second option creates the impression that you may have actually read some landmark papers and drawn your own conclusions on their content. Such papers as MAGPIE, ENIGMA 1 and POISE are just a few of a number of landmark papers in recent years. Important papers are referenced at the end of each marking plan and we would recommend you have a look at them. It is quite acceptable to drop the year of publication followed by either the title or principal author into your answer.

## Should I use abbreviations and acronyms?

Abbrevs. are usfl. tm'svrs. but can b. pot. annoying. They therefore need to be used sensibly. The first encounter should be as full text (unless its use is very widespread such as INR) followed by the shorter version in brackets. After that it would be acceptable to use the abbreviation or acronym throughout your answer.

## Are handwriting, spelling and grammar important?

It is now quite reasonable for an examiner to withhold some of the 2 marks out of 20 assigned for each question for clarity, judgement and the ability to prioritise if the presentation is poor. You will be allowed a certain amount of poor handwriting as the examiner understands that you are writing under extreme conditions. If, however, your writing is deteriorating to the point where it is making the examiner's work difficult to extract meaning from your text, then you may lose marks. In extreme cases we have known of high-quality candidates failing the exam and, on appeal, when their paper was reviewed it was widely agreed to be illegible.

Poor spelling and grammar may potentially annoy the examiner. Some will be more pernickety than others. This may come as a shock to you but an examiner will not scrutinise every word of every answer you write. What poor spelling and grammar may do is alert the examiner to the fact (often incorrectly) that you are a weaker candidate. This is a bad thing to do as they will scrutinise your work closely and may choose to not give you the benefit of the doubt on an answer where you are mainly right. Do whatever you can to avoid annoying the examiners. Writing, spelling and grammar assessment is another very good reason to do some practice papers under exam conditions and show them to a senior colleague.

## Is it essential to stick to time?

Yes! This is very important. Let us consider the circumstances under which you might be tempted to spread the time unevenly. You look at the paper and notice a question in an area in which you are very strong and another where you feel you are pretty clueless. You think that you might write a cursory answer for the difficult question ensuring a '1' mark, and try to make that up by writing a 28 minute answer in your strong area to achieve a '2+'. This averages you out to the equivalent of a '1 +, 2' performance and would keep you in the game. The problem here is that it is much more difficult to predictably convert a 2 to a 2+ than a 1 to a 1+ or even a 2. You have to hit the examiner's marking sheet with most of the essential and desirable content to get near a '2+'. Most questions that you think you are clueless on will unravel during the 15-minute writing process and you will get plenty of good-quality content. This especially goes for non-clinical questions that may initially look daunting. A little thought and organisation will often allow you to mine a rich vein of content.

## How much should I write per question?

Different people write different amounts with a wide range of precision and content in 15 minutes. You must find out what you are capable of. This is another good reason for using this book because it may be evident after a few essays that you have the wrong approach. There are a few generalisations that can be made. Content is king. You have to put enough correct content down to score a threshold mark to pass a question. This is unavoidable. It is difficult, unless you are unfeasibly succinct, to record enough content in fewer than 100 words. In general, essays we see on the Crammer with 40–80 words are written by the weaker candidates and lack content. They almost invariably score low. If following a practice paper you realise that you are only writing 65 words per 15-minute essay, then there are two likely explanations. First, you did not know enough to write more. This has an easy solution, which is learn more. Second, you may have known plenty, but were unable to write more in 15 minutes. This may occur throughout the paper or as fatigue sets in towards the end. This also has a simple solution and that is practice writing loads more essays.

On the upper end, we will see candidates on the course write 300–350 words in 15 minutes. If this is your style, your answers are content-heavy, well structured, consistent throughout the paper and do not run over time, then I would not discourage you from this practice. However, we will often find that the high scores on any given essay may be the ones with a 120-word answer ramming all the point-scoring content in succinctly. High-word-count essays usually run to three or four sides of A4. It is often the case that there will be half-side patches that score absolutely zero as the candidate may be off the point or writing a long-winded introductory paragraph. This is time wasted that should be spent firing down content elsewhere. Overblown, wordy answers will also not help you score the 2 extra points per essay allocated for clarity, judgement and the ability to prioritise.

## How should I divide my time within one question with multiple parts?

Since October 2004, the College has shown the percentage marks available for each part of a question. Broadly allow 1 minute per 10% of marks. Be vigilant on questions such as:

'A patient on the ICU, who had cardiac surgery completed 3 hours ago, is still intubated.

a) What clinical features might suggest the development of acute cardiac tamponade? (55%)
b) How might you confirm the diagnosis? (5%)
c) Outline your management of acute cardiac tamponade? (40%)' (*from Oct 2004.*)

To waste more than a sentence or two on part b) would be inappropriate, even if it is the subject of your PhD thesis.

## How do I deal with my own irrelevant thoughts

Sometimes on first appearance a question may fire off a multitude of thoughts in your brain; it is important to try to keep your answer relevant to the question. A good discipline is to ask yourself 'What does this question include and what does it exclude?' This means that, for instance, if you receive the question 'Describe the features of the anaesthetic machine which are intended to prevent the delivery of a hypoxic mixture to the patient' (*Oct 2001*), it is only about hypoxic mixture and not about other safety features. It is also about the whole anaesthetic machine including everything from pipelines to the common gas outlet. This momentary check will stop you wasting time with irrelevancies and stop you missing important areas of content.

## What should I do if a question is 'dodgy'?

Every once in a while a question appears in The Final which is ambiguous or contentious. This is a rare occurrence but does still happen. Our advice if you are concerned about a question is to carry on writing but raise your hand. Ask the examiner about your area of concern. Do not get into a heated discussion, but make your concerns known. Examiners have to log all enquiries during the exam. If enough people raise concerns about a given question it will be reviewed and may be removed from the final marks. This process should waste as little of your time as possible and it is vital that you still write an answer. Try to cover most bases superficially.

Diplomatically point out ambiguities or contentious areas when phrasing your answer.

## What happens if I turn the paper over and I see an unanswerable question?

This is the nightmare that most Final FRCA candidates have at some point. You wake up having just imagined turning the paper over to find 'What are the special features that need to be considered when preparing to intubate someone with Bonzini's syndrome?' The reality is that this will not happen. If you have revised in anything like a sensible and diligent way, you will be able to start writing something for all the questions. It is not in the College's interest to put esoteric questions into the exam as they do not test the field effectively and they may have to remove the question from consideration. It is a common nightmare, but it will not happen. Revise hard and sleep easy.

## What happens if I turn the paper over and I see a very difficult question?

Difficult questions do crop up. In October 2002, the College asked the question 'Define contractility. Outline the methods available to the clinician to assess myocardial contractility in the perioperative period'. At the time this was thought to be a particularly tough question unless it fell into your area of sub-specialist knowledge. The heartening thought when presented with such a question is that if you have revised sensibly, across a broad area of the syllabus, then if you think a question is difficult it is extremely likely that most other people sitting the paper will also find that question difficult. You therefore need to get as much relevant content down in the 15 minutes for that question in the knowledge that most other people in the exam room are in the same position. Some will not respond in such a calm way and will not hit as many content points as you. Make definitions, classify where possible and apply some structure to your answer. For example, in the above question on contractility, a clinical assessment of the patient looking at perfusion and examining the minimal mandatory monitoring will give a basic assessment of contractility. This should be mentioned and put into the context of other factors that influence cardiac output, before moving on to the more complex assessment techniques. Quite often stating the obvious and applying a sensible classification system will score you a healthy amount of points.

## Is it true that they usually start with an easy first question?

This was a rumour a few years ago and had even been presented to us as a negative problem. Candidates felt that the College were putting a straightforward clinical question in at the beginning and people were spending beyond their allotted 15 minutes on territory on which they felt comfortable. This immediately put them behind the clock and led to timing problems. Shortly after this came to the surface, a couple of papers with real stinkers for first questions came along, dispelling this rumour. However, the learning point is still there and it is that you must stick to time with an almost religious fervour.

## What happens if I find myself with 25 minutes left with three questions to do?

If you've followed the advice in this book, you can discount this particular nightmare as, with good discipline, this should never happen to you. Let's say that you got particularly carried away on the day of the exam and spent too long on a question. You now find yourself with the scenario above. What to do? Well, first, don't panic. Your discipline now needs to be even better than normal. You are exhausted with hand cramp and a reduced time per question. You must allocate even time to the remaining questions. Just over 8 minutes per question is all you should allow yourself. Try to hit the main points of the question. Leave out the minutiae if it means you will run out of time hitting the main points in the second part of your answer. Go for lists and bullet points wherever possible. Get as much relevant, good-quality content down as possible. Do not, under any circumstances, fail to give any of the three remaining questions 8 minutes of your time. In 8 minutes, there should be plenty of content that will score heavily. Remember, to fail to write an answer is immediate failure in the whole exam.

## What's the best way to revise?

Sorry, but we do not have the perfect answer to this question. What is clear is that different people have different ways of effectively revising. Some people will sit down for 6-hour stints with a pack of biscuits and read Miller cover to cover four times in the run up to the exam. Other people will use a large number of small books and read in 20-minute bursts. If you are good at one of these two tactics, stick with it. Remember that The Final is founded on the knowledge gained in Primary. It is therefore a good idea in the first place to look over your notes from the Primary Examination. This is also the reason why, in general, we will encourage candidates to avoid postponing the Final Examination. The closer you are to your Primary knowledge base, the fresher it will be in your mind. Having a feel for the size of the task in hand will also help effective revision. To tackle the full syllabus it helps if you first understand what the syllabus might be. The College publishes a syllabus in its examination section for basic and intermediate training. This is a good starting point. Surveillance of topic areas arising in practice MCQs and SAQs will help to supplement this. Ticking covered areas off will help to build your confidence that you are getting through the vast pile of work required. A frequently quoted statement is that 'There is an unavoidable truth that you have to chew a certain amount of cardboard to pass The Final FRCA'. The College through its CPD supplements to the BJA and the Association through its published pamphlets provide an invaluable source of text that is current, topical and written by experts. Every candidate attempting The Final should make sure they have read all of these publications for the last 5 years.

The final point on revision that we would like to cover is the usefulness of reading journals. Two of us regularly lecture on Final FRCA courses on 'Current Topics in Anaesthesia'. The preparation for this involves, amongst other things, reviewing the content of the main anaesthetic journals for the last year. What is always interesting is that when you look across a number of journals such as *BJA, Anaesthesia, Anesthesiology* and *Anesthesia and Analgesia*, in the space of a year, a lot of topics are covered in most of the journals in editorials or review articles. A quick glance at these topics indicates that they represent the cutting edge of the syllabus. In the last few years, topics such as recombinant factor VIIa or ICU care bundles had been covered by most journals in a fairly short period after they became news. It doesn't stretch the imagination too far to imagine how this process occurs at editorial meetings. This means that journals are great source material for syllabus-relevant, up-to-date topics. The problem is that journals always appear large and full of irrelevant papers on rodent psychology or advertising. There is a skill to extracting the useful content out of journals in the most efficient way. Editorials and review articles in the table of contents should be assessed for potential quality information. Other papers in the journal can also be quickly appraised. If a paper is about an area that has some relevance to the syllabus, it might be worth a look at the abstract and introduction. Even if a whole paper itself is not useful, the introduction may be. For example, in a paper about postoperative nausea and vomiting with sufentanil use in day case surgery, you may work in a country where sufentanil is not available. The results of the study may not be of much use to you, but the introduction may contain some helpful information about postoperative nausea and vomiting in day case surgery. The journals may also act as an alternative to the books when you are approaching the end of revision and feeling a bit stale. Their contemporary nature can often feel quite refreshing in the final run up to the exam.

The website www.frca.co.uk also has lots of useful resources worth having a look at leading up to the exam. The same can also be said for the College Final FRCA book.

We would also advise, where possible, for you to get together with other people sitting the exam and organise yourselves into study groups. These can involve, for example, such activities as doing MCQs together, marking each other's practice SAQs or each taking on difficult topics and explaining them to the rest of the group.

## How should I use this book?

This book may be used in a number of ways. The nine papers are presented in a style that mimics the real paper set by the College with twelve 15-minute questions. We would encourage you to sit down and attempt at least one of these papers in as close to exam conditions as you can simulate. Sit at a desk with a pad of paper and pen. Ensure no interruptions for 3 hours. Have a clock on the wall. Do not look at the paper beforehand. Sit down and turn the paper over, noting the time. Start at Question 1 and spend 15 minutes answering. At exactly 15 minutes into your mock exam, move on to Question 2. Carry on for 3 hours.

Many things can be gained from this exercise. When we ask on The Crammer Course how many people have sat down and written a whole 3-hour paper in preparation for this exam, usually fewer than 15% of first-time sitters answer yes. This is the equivalent of turning up to the London Marathon having done a few 3-mile runs. This makes little sense. It is one of the great recurring tragedies of the exam year in year out. Excellent candidates come up to visit after the paper and say how they knew stuff but in the last few questions just couldn't write enough down. This is usually presented as 'I ran out of time' but on further questioning it is usually apparent that they ran out of time because they were slowly and painfully fighting the hand cramps at the end to scratch down low-word-count answers with a claw-like grasp on their pens. After a recent paper, a candidate told me that for the last three questions her writing had gone into VT.

Having a go at the whole paper lets you know what you are up against and lets you pace yourself earlier on by, for example, choosing a bulleted list rather than a longer paragraph of text. It may help you make a very simple improvement by identifying that you are using the wrong pen. That favourite ballpen you use to write down your seagulls on an anaesthetic chart may require a bit too much downward pressure for a 3-hour essay paper. We recommend candidates try the gel pens that only require a very light touch to make a mark. Buy three or four new ones just for the exam. (If this makes the difference you'll still be more than £650 up.) Changing to a new pen may be a nice little pick-me-up in the middle of the exam, like a tennis player changing their shirt between sets (the shirt-changing activity is generally frowned upon by the College). Getting your pen right may seem unnecessary attention to detail, but if it helps you cram your answers with a bit more content and punts your mark up by just 1%, this can have a dramatic effect on passing the exam. Remember that most of you reading this book will be grouped close to the mean on a normal distribution curve for your marks in this exam. If, within that population, the group who take 'Correct pen advice' move by 1% to the right in the normal distribution, a large number of you will cross the pass-mark threshold. Small margin improvements make a big difference in this exam for the main body of candidates. Small adjustments that individually produce small gains will also combine to give that extra few per cent that may make all the difference.

In the answer section to this book we have endeavoured to produce a model answer to give you a feel for a standard. We are not examiners at the College but, through running the Crammer Course and tutoring trainees, we have a good idea of the standard required. The book can therefore also be used to see how your performance rates against a standard. We have set up the marking scheme in accordance with the College's latest information. College tutors or education supervisors may want to sit their trainees down and give them a go at sitting a full or part paper, then take the answers away and mark against the model answers. It should be noted that sometimes, especially when a list is asked for that may be extensive, and only a low percentage of the marks are available, it may be that the model answer is longer than would be recommended in the real exam. Where possible we will try to indicate this in the 'Additional Notes' for the question. These also exist at the beginning of many of the answers to give specific advice or comment about an individual essay.

We have tried to indicate, where possible, the parts of answers that are 'Essential', 'Desirable' and 'Supplementary' by marking with two($\star\star$), one($\star$) or no stars() respectively.

If formally using the book to mark a paper, the allocation of points for each section of an individual question is the percentage marks for that section divided by 5 to get a mark out of 20.

Compared to the model answer, score the given answer allowing points for total content and prioritisation of essential information over desirable information over supplementary information.

As a guide, an answer with all the essential information and some desirable information would score 50% of the available points.

At the end of the question add up all the sections to give a score out of 18. 0, 1 or 2 points should then be added for clarity, judgement and the ability to prioritise. This is why the percentages for each question only add up to 90%.

If the answer contains serious errors more than 2 points may be withheld but reasons for this must be given.

A representative guide as to what would be a pass or 2+ pass is difficult to quantify as it varies from question to question and paper to paper. On our course, generally 9–14 scores a 2, and 15 or greater scores a 2+.

Finally the book can be used to aid revision of certain key topics. The choice of questions were at the time of press all questions that we thought fulfilled the criteria of being relevant, contemporary and testing widespread, non-controversial, evidence-based topic areas. We have tried where possible to include references or URLs which direct the reader to source material or further reading.

*Good luck!*
*(We all need some sometimes.)*
*Dr James Nickells*
*Dr Andy Georgiou*
*Dr Ben Walton*

# Question Papers

# Paper 1

Three hour paper. Answer all the questions.
Where we have indicated the way marks are allocated, candidates are advised to spend their time accordingly.
10% of the marks for each question would be awarded for clarity, judgement and the ability to prioritise; marks would be deducted for serious errors.

## Question 1

a) Illustrate the anatomy of the femoral triangle and its contents. (35%)
b) List the indications for a 'three-in-one block'. (20%)
c) How would you perform a fascia iliacus block? (35%)

## Question 2

What are the specific problems in the anaesthetic management of a patient with acromegaly undergoing transphenoidal hypophysectomy? (90%)

## Question 3

a) A fit 28-year-old primigravida with an uncomplicated pregnancy of 39 weeks gestation is in labour and has a cervical dilatation of 8cm. She rapidly becomes breathless and collapses with a weak pulse. What is the differential diagnosis? (30%)
b) What clinical features would suggest that the diagnosis is one of amniotic fluid embolus? (30%)
c) What would be your immediate management of this patient? (30%)

## Question 4

a) What factors increase the risk of intraoperative aspiration of abdominal contents? (45%)
b) How would you reduce the risk of significant aspiration in the perioperative period? (45%)

## Question 5

An anxious 54-year-old lady requires a laparotomy for large bowel obstruction under general anaesthesia. At the preoperative visit she informs you that she is currently involved in litigation following a period of awareness under anaesthesia for haemorrhoidectomy.

Summarise the points you would raise in the preoperative discussion in relation to awareness and her proposed anaesthetic. (90%)

## Question 6

a) List the complications of blood transfusion that may occur within the operating theatre. (50%)
b) Outline the steps that need to be taken to ensure a unit of packed red cells received by the patient is the correct one. (40%)

## Question 7

a) How do you select an appropriately sized blood pressure cuff for a patient? (10%)
b) What are the principles behind the non-invasive methods of blood pressure measurement? (40%)
c) The measurement of invasive blood pressure requires a transducer. What is a transducer and what is its mechanism of action in this context? (40%)

## Question 8

A 46-year-old 95kg previously healthy patient is brought into the emergency department having been extricated from a burning car by the fire brigade following a motor vehicle collision. He has burns to the face and significant circumferential burns to the torso and upper limbs and the GCS was recorded as 13.

a) What in particular would you be looking for during your initial survey of this patient? (35%)
b) What intraoperative problems might you predict were this patient to be taken to theatre for debridement of his burns? (40%)
c) List the drugs you would have drawn up at induction, 3 hours after the vehicle accident, giving the doses you would expect to administer. (15%)

## Question 9

a) What is your choice of crystalloid for intravenous intraoperative fluid replacement in paediatric anaesthesia? Outline why some fluids are less suitable than your first choice. (50%)
b) How would you calculate the maintenance fluid regimen for a child? (20%)
c) Why might you fluid-restrict a sick child? (20%)

## Question 10

Define the following:
a) Nociception. (10%)
b) Allodynia. (10%)
c) Hyperalgesia. (10%)
d) Neuropathic pain. (10%)
e) What is the mechanism of action of gabapentin and when might it be useful in the management of chronic pain? (50%)

## Question 11

Three weeks prior to admission for laparoscopic right hemicolectomy for carcinoma a 77-year-old patient attends a pre-assessment clinic. He has ischaemic heart disease, heart failure, smokes and gets short of breath after walking 50 metres on flat, level ground.

a) List the advantages of seeing this gentleman 6 weeks prior to surgery. (30%)
b) At this appointment and from subsequent investigations how could he be assessed and then, up to the day before admission, optimised for surgery? (60%)

## Question 12

a) What are the indications for commencing total parenteral nutrition in a ventilated patient on intensive care? (20%)
b) How would you determine a patient's daily calorie requirement? (20%)
c) Outline the uses of lipid emulsion in anaesthesia and critical care. (50%)

# Paper 2

Three hour paper. Answer all the questions.
Where we have indicated the way marks are allocated, candidates are advised to spend their time accordingly.
10% of the marks for each question would be awarded for clarity, judgement and the ability to prioritise; marks would be deducted for serious errors.

## Question 1

a) Draw a transverse section through the axilla at the level of the inferior border of the pectoralis major at its humeral insertion, detailing the anatomical relations of the axillary artery and the brachial plexus. (50%)
b) List the surgical indications for supraclavicular blockade of the brachial plexus. (10%)
c) List the potential complications of an interscalene block. (30%)

## Question 2

a) Briefly outline the treatment options for weight reduction available to a patient with Class III obesity (BMI >40). (60%)
b) When anaesthetising this patient, how would you optimise oxygenation and position the patient for intubation prior to induction? (30%)

## Question 3

a) Draw a labelled schematic diagram of a co-axial Mapleson D anaesthetic breathing system showing fresh gas flow entering the system. (30%)
b) Why is a Mapleson D inefficient for spontaneous ventilation yet efficient for intermittent positive pressure ventilation (IPPV)? (30%)
c) Give two advantages and disadvantages of a co-axial D over an unmodified system. (10%)
d) Give two ways that one can check that the inner lumen of a coaxial D (Bain) is safe to use. (20%)

## Question 4

What are the special considerations required when anaesthetising a patient with carcinoid syndrome for removal of a gastric tumour? (90%)

# Question 5

In patients with chronic liver disease undergoing anaesthesia:

a) What are the relevant physiological changes which must be considered? (60%)
b) What pharmacological considerations affect the choice of neuromuscular blocker? (30%)

# Question 6

a) Give a definition of delirium as applied to a patient on a critical care unit. (10%)
b) List the causes of delirium in a patient on a critical care unit. (40%)
c) How may the incidence of delirium be kept to a minimum in a critical care unit? (40%)

# Question 7

a) What are the clinical features of critical illness polyneuropathy (CIPN)? (30%)
b) List the predisposing factors. (20%).
c) How is it diagnosed? (20%)
d) What are the difficulties encountered when managing a ventilated, critically ill patient with this condition? (20%)

# Question 8

a) Draw a waveform one would expect to see when transducing a central venous catheter inserted into an ASA 1 patient with a structurally normal heart. Explain which parts of the cardiac cycle cause the various undulations on this waveform. On the same diagram draw an ECG tracing showing the temporal relationship between the two. (30%)
b) List the factors that increase and decrease the central venous pressure. (20%)
c) What information can be gained from digital examination of an arterial pulse? (40%)

# Question 9

a) What are the cardiovascular effects of pregnancy at full term? (60%)
b) What physical manoeuvres can be performed to optimise cardiovascular function at the beginning of an elective caesarean section under regional anaesthesia? (30%)

# Question 10

a) With the aid of the schematic diagram of a nephron show where the following classes of diuretic act, giving an example of each and briefly outline their mechanism of action.

Loop diuretic (10%)
Osmotic diuretic (10%)
Thiazide diuretic (10%)
Potassium sparing diuretic (10%)
Carbonic anhydrase inhibitor (10%)

See Figure 1.

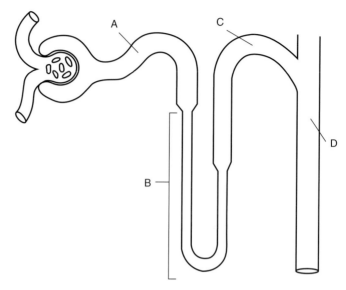

A Schematic Drawing of a Nephron

Figure 1

b) Discuss the potential risks associated with anaesthetising patients taking diuretics. (40%)

## Question 11

a) List the ideal physicochemical properties of a volatile agent for use in the gaseous induction of anaesthesia. (30%)
b) Why is a gaseous induction in an 18-month-old child more rapid than one in an adult? (30%)
c) Why may upper airway obstruction slow this process? (30%)

## Question 12

a) What is Parkinson's disease? (30%)
b) A 68-year-old male patient with Parkinson's disease is medicated with co-beneldopa (levodopa/benserazide) and cabergoline. He is scheduled for a laparoscopic cholecystectomy. What are the anaesthetic considerations specific to this patient? (60%)

# Paper 3

Three hour paper. Answer all the questions.
Where we have indicated the way marks are allocated, candidates are advised to spend their time accordingly.
10% of the marks for each question would be awarded for clarity, judgement and the ability to prioritise; marks would be deducted for serious errors.

## Question 1

a) What are the anatomical relations of the tracheal carina? (50%)
b) List the indications for one-lung ventilation. (30%)
c) List the methods available for one-lung ventilation. (10%)

## Question 2

After induction of anaesthesia in a 75kg adult for a routine case you discover that you cannot intubate or ventilate the patient. You have given 7mg of vecuronium at induction. A laryngeal mask airway (LMA) is not helpful. Describe what you would do next. (90%)

## Question 3

a) How does an intra-aortic balloon pump exert its physiological action and when might it be used? (45%)
b) What may be the reasons for a patient failing to wean from cardiopulmonary bypass following coronary artery bypass grafting? (45%)

## Question 4

What measures would you employ to minimise the risk of central venous catheter (CVC) related infection in an intensive care unit you work in? (90%)

## Question 5

a) What pathological factors make a patient unsuitable for day case (12 hour stay)? (50%)
b) Discuss the use of regional anaesthesia in day case. (40%)

## Question 6

a) You are called to the emergency department to see a 40-year-old patient known to have taken an overdose of amitriptyline. What clinical features are consistent with an overdose of this nature? (40%)
b) In an adult patient with a history of paracetamol overdose, what investigations would you perform to determine the significance of the overdose (20%) and to monitor the patient's condition? (30%)

## Question 7

a) The administration of multiple drugs in a short space of time means that anaesthetists are likely to make drug errors. How can this risk be reduced in the setting of a day case surgery unit? (40%)
b) How might the safety of epidural drug delivery for labour be improved? (50%)

## Question 8

a) Briefly outline the uses of a fibreoptic bronchoscope in anaesthetic practice. (45%)
b) Once used for a percutaneous tracheostomy, describe the process by which the bronchoscope is made ready to be used again. (45%)

## Question 9

An 18-year-old girl is ventilated on ITU two days following a road traffic accident during which she sustained a significant head injury (depressed skull fracture, bifrontal contusions and an extradural haematoma that has been evacuated). She has a cerebrospinal fluid (CSF) drain in and her intracranial pressure (ICP) has been stable but in the last hour it has risen from 10 to 30mmHg.

a) Why might this have occurred? (40%)
b) What sequence of management would you institute? (50%)

## Question 10

a) How may humidity be defined? (20%)
b) List the devices used to measure humidity, describing the working principles of one of these in detail. (50%)
c) What is the clinical relevance of ensuring an appropriate level of humidity is obtained in the environment of a patient? (20%)

## Question 11

a) What physiological changes occur when a patient is placed in the prone position? (30%)
b) What are the complications of anaesthesia in the prone position? (60%)

## Question 12

Classically, a new drug will undergo four phases of clinical trials in humans.

a) Briefly outline the purpose of each of these phases. (40%)
   The Committee on Safety of Medicines produces a yellow card to be submitted in the event of an adverse drug reaction.
b) Under what circumstances would you fill in a yellow card? (50%)

# Paper 4

Three hour paper. Answer all the questions.
Where we have indicated the way marks are allocated, candidates are advised to spend their time accordingly.
10% of the marks for each question would be awarded for clarity, judgement and the ability to prioritise; marks would be deducted for serious errors.

## Question 1

When a person donates a 'pint of blood' this is converted into a number of different blood products.

a) What are these products, what are they usually stored in and at what temperatures? (30%)
b) State what is contained in cryoprecipitate and list transfusion triggers for platelet transfusion. (20%)
c) How is a crossmatch carried out in the laboratory? (40%)

## Question 2

a) List the factors leading to a delay in the start of a theatre list. (40%)
b) How might the efficiency of a theatre list be improved? (50%)

## Question 3

a) What is digoxin and what are the indications for its use? (15%)
b) What is the mechanism of action of digoxin? (30%)
c) A 55-year-old patient is scheduled for an open right hemicolectomy. How might the preoperative discovery of atrial fibrillation on the ECG change your approach to this patient's anaesthetic? (45%)

## Question 4

Concerning Do Not Attempt to Resuscitate orders (DNAR orders):

a) Discuss reasons why a DNAR order may be implemented. (40%)
An intellectually high-performing (IQ 135) 14-year-old with severe spasticity from cerebral palsy attending for contracture release has stated that should she have a cardiac arrest under anaesthesia she wishes not to be resuscitated. Her parents are adamant she should be.

b) What are the specific issues that you would wish to clarify in your preoperative discussions and who else would you involve with specific reference to this issue? (50%)

## Question 5

Describe the mechanism of action of the agents which may be used to artificially elevate gastric pH. (90%)

## Question 6

a) How is lactate produced in the human body? (40%)
b) What are the causes of a lactic acidosis? (50%)

## Question 7

a) Draw the view obtained during direct laryngoscopy of a Cormack and Lehane Grade 1 intubation. (40%)
b) List the possible causes and differential diagnosis of laryngospasm. (20%)
c) At the end of a case following removal of the endotracheal tube a 4-year-old child appears to go into laryngospasm. Outline your management strategy. (30%)

## Question 8

a) What are the physical differences between a re-usable laryngeal mask and an intubating laryngeal mask (iLMA)? (20%)
b) What are the indications for using an iLMA? (20%)
c) What would you do if your first attempt to intubate down an iLMA were unsuccessful? (50%)

## Question 9

a) What criteria must be met for a patient to be considered for a Non-Heart-Beating Organ Donation (NHBD)? (25%)
b) Describe a timeline for an intensive care patient being considered for NHBD through to organ retrieval. (40%)
c) What advantages does beating-heart donation have over NHBD? (25%)

## Question 10

a) What are the mechanisms bacteria use to gain resistance to antibiotics? (40%)
b) What clinical problems are typically caused by vancomycin-resistant enterococci (VRE) and what antibiotics would you use to treat a sick patient found to have VRE bacteraemia? (50%)

## Question 11

A woman who is 36 weeks pregnant and from out of area presents at 4 a.m. to the delivery suite complaining of low abdominal pain and vaginal bleeding for 4 hours. She also reports being told she has a 'low-lying placenta'. The obstetric registrar on call asks for your help.

a) Describe your initial assessment of the patient. (30%)
b) Draw a table displaying the severity of the blood loss and common physiological variables. (20%)

The obstetrician tells you that there are signs of fetal distress and that they would like to proceed to delivery by caesarean section.

c) Describe your anaesthetic management of this case. (40%)

## Question 12

a) How would you identify a patient at risk of postoperative nausea and vomiting (PONV)? (40%)

b) What preventive measures do you take to reduce the chance of PONV? (50%)

# Paper 5

Three hour paper. Answer all the questions.
Where we have indicated the way marks are allocated, candidates are advised to spend their time accordingly.
10% of the marks for each question would be awarded for clarity, judgement and the ability to prioritise; marks would be deducted for serious errors.

## Question 1

a) What are the difficulties encountered when managing acute pain in a patient with pre-existing opioid dependence? (40%)
b) How can optimum analgesia be provided for these patients? (50%)

## Question 2

a) Illustrate the anatomy of the circle of Willis. (50%)
b) Describe its physiological importance and the reasons for potential failure of this system. (40%)

## Question 3

a) Plastic surgeons often get concerned when performing a free flap operation that the flap may become ischaemic. How might this ischaemia occur? (40%)
b) How, as an anaesthetist, can one ensure that a free flap has the best chance of maintaining adequate perfusion in the intraoperative period? (50%)

## Question 4

A 36-year-old woman who has Graves disease presents to the Emergency Department with a cold, pulseless arm of sudden onset. Over the last 3 months she has lost 12 pounds, and developed a hoarse voice. Examination is remarkable for a fine tremor and an obvious goitre. Observations: HR 118/min (irregularly irregular), BP 143/92, temp 37.8°C.

The vascular surgeons wish to perform a CT angiogram and get her to theatre as soon as possible.

a) How would you evaluate her airway preoperatively? (30%)
b) What are the specific risks associated with anaesthetising a patient with hyperthyroidism? (30%)
c) What drugs would you use to treat her hyperthyroidism? Give a brief description of how each drug exerts its effect. (30%)

## Question 5

You are asked to anaesthetise a 32-year-old male for incision and drainage of a groin abscess. He is known to be HIV-positive. Outline the features of your preoperative clinical assessment of this patient that specifically relate to HIV. (90%)

## Question 6

a) What are the consequences of intraoperative hypothermia? (40%)
b) Briefly outline the mechanisms by which heat is lost in the anaesthetised patient. (25%)
c) By what means may intraoperative heat loss be minimised? (25%)

## Question 7

a) How should a patient be correctly monitored at induction and during maintenance of general anaesthesia for a high saphenous ligation, strip and avulsions? (50%)
b) What may cause inaccuracies when measuring oxygen saturation using a pulse oximeter? (40%)

## Question 8

a) What are the potential advantages and disadvantages of a critical care outreach team? (45%)
b) In 2007 the National Institute for Clinical Excellence (NICE) published a document 'Acutely Ill Patients in Hospital'. Outline its main recommendations. (45%)

## Question 9

a) What are the risk factors for development of post-dural-puncture headache (PDPH)? (40%)
   A woman who received an epidural as part of her pain relief during labour develops a headache 6 hours post-delivery, after the epidural catheter has been removed.
b) List the differential diagnoses of her headache. (10%)
c) If this turns out to be a PDPH, outline your subsequent management. (40%)

## Question 10

a) List the potential advantages of percutaneous tracheostomy over prolonged endotracheal intubation in a patient ventilated on critical care. (50%)
b) How would you assess whether a patient is safe to have their tracheostomy removed (decannulated)? (40%)

## Question 11

a) What characteristics set remifentanil apart from other opioid analgesics and why? (40%)
b) What problems are common to all sedative agents within a critical care setting? (20%)
c) What are the potential advantages of switching from a hypnotic-based sedative regime to an analgesic-based sedation regime using remifentanil? (30%)

## Question 12

What are the special considerations when anaesthetising a patient with probable variant CJD requiring gamma-nailing of a fractured femur? (90%)

# Paper 6

Three hour paper. Answer all the questions.
Where we have indicated the way marks are allocated, candidates are advised to spend their time accordingly.
10% of the marks for each question would be awarded for clarity, judgement and the ability to prioritise; marks would be deducted for serious errors.

## Question 1

a) Describe the anatomy of the coeliac plexus. (40%)
b) What are the indications for coeliac plexus blockade? (10%)
c) How is blockade of the coeliac plexus performed? (40%)

## Question 2

A 72-year-old male patient is undergoing an open reduction and internal fixation of the right ankle under general anaesthesia following a fall 1 day previously. Thirty minutes after the start of surgery, you notice ST elevation on the ECG.

a) What is your immediate management? (45%)
b) How would you proceed in light of persisting ST elevation once the wound is closed? (45%)

## Question 3

What investigations should be performed on a patient suspected to have had an anaphylactic reaction under an anaesthetic you administered? (90%)

## Question 4

A 46-year-old woman is listed for a laparoscopic cholecystectomy as a day case. She weighs 113 kilos and is 150cm in height. What anaesthetic challenges does this case present? (90%)

## Question 5

An otherwise fit and well 52-year-old woman presents for surgery for acoustic neuroma. The surgeon informs you that this is a technically difficult case which he anticipates taking 10 to 12 hours. What are the problems and what specific measures would you take when anaesthetising such a long operation? (90%)

# Question 6

a) The oxygen saturation in the left ventricle of a fetus is 65%. List the physiological mechanisms that allow the fetus to tolerate this degree of relative hypoxaemia. (40%)
b) What pharmacokinetic differences between adults and neonates are relevant to anaesthesia? (50%)

# Question 7

a) What markings are present on the valve block and body of an oxygen cylinder? State where these markings are (cylinder body or valve block). (50%)
b) For transfer of a 70kg intubated and fully ventilated patient on a journey anticipated to take 120 minutes, calculate how much oxygen you would take to ensure safe transfer. Show your calculations and assumptions. Give your answer in litres and number of 'E'-sized cylinders. (40%)

# Question 8

a) What are the symptoms and signs of a right-sided pleural effusion? (30%)
b) State how pleural effusions can be classified and give examples of each. (20%)
c) What tests need to be performed on a sample of pleural fluid to identify the nature of the effusion? (40%)

# Question 9

a) What are the patient risk factors that are known to influence surgical risk? (50%)
b) List the physiological variables required to calculate a P-POSSUM score. (40%)

# Question 10

a) What is pre-eclampsia and how is it diagnosed? (20%)
b) List the effects of pre-eclampsia on maternal physiology. (30%)
c) Describe the principles of management of a patient with pre-eclampsia, giving examples. (40%)

# Question 11

a) What are the indications for inserting a spinal cord stimulator? (50%)
b) What are the complications of this procedure? (40%)

# Question 12

a) What devices are available to deliver drugs to a patient transdermally? (20%)
b) What factors influence the systemic uptake of transdermally applied drugs? (40%)
c) How can the uptake of transdermally applied drugs be increased? (30%)

# Paper 7

Three hour paper. Answer all the questions.
Where we have indicated the way marks are allocated, candidates are advised to spend their time accordingly.
10% of the marks for each question would be awarded for clarity, judgement and the ability to prioritise; marks would be deducted for serious errors.

## Question 1

a) How is $CO_2$ transported in arterial and venous blood? (20%)
b) Illustrate graphically how the $CO_2$ content of blood varies with $PaCO_2$. (15%)
c) Why is $CO_2$ transport better in deoxygenated than oxygenated blood? (25%)
d) What does sodalime contain and how does it eliminate $CO_2$ from a circle system? (30%)

## Question 2

a) How would you classify recreational drugs? Give three examples in each class. (25%)
b) How would you classify controlled drugs? (15%)
c) What are your responsibilities as an anaesthetist when handling controlled drugs? (50%)

## Question 3

a) Draw a transverse section through the spinal cord at the level of the third cervical vertebra (C3) showing the ascending and descending neural pathways. (50%)
b) Describe the symptoms and signs which may result from:
   – a unilateral cord lesion in the thoracic spine at the level of the fourth thoracic vertebra (T4). (20%)
   – a complete transverse cord lesion in the thoracic spine at T4. (20%)

## Question 4

a) What is the physiological role of magnesium in the body? (30%)
b) List the indications for the use of magnesium as a therapeutic agent. (30%)
c) What are the harmful effects of magnesium therapy which may be seen in the context of anaesthesia? (30%)

# Question 5

a) Briefly describe how an image is generated by a magnetic resonance imaging (MRI) scanner. (45%)
b) What are the particular difficulties in anaesthetising a patient within an MRI scanner that are different from those in other remote locations? (45%)

# Question 6

a) What risk factors put a patient at risk of developing methicillin-resistant *Staphylococcus aureus* (MRSA) infection during a stay in hospital? (30%)
b) What preventive measures have been shown to be effective in minimising the spread of MRSA within a hospital? (60%)

# Question 7

a) What is the role of the National Institute for Clinical Excellence (NICE) and how does it develop a clinical guideline? (50%)
b) Name a recent NICE report that is of direct clinical relevance to anaesthetists or critical care doctors and outline the main findings. (40%)

# Question 8

a) Briefly describe the World Health Organization's (WHO) pain-relief ladder. (30%)
b) What cautions and contraindications are there to the prescription of non-steroidal anti-inflammatory drugs (NSAIDs)? (20%)
c) What advantages does a 1g dose of intravenous paracetamol have over a 1g oral dose of paracetamol when administered to an adult patient after general anaesthesia for four third molar extractions? (40%)

# Question 9

a) What advice would you give a 35-year-old patient who is 8 weeks pregnant with acute appendicitis requiring surgery, when she asks you 'Will the anaesthetic affect my baby?' (40%)
b) A patient is 32 weeks into an uncomplicated pregnancy and develops acute, severe, neurological signs and symptoms requiring an urgent lumbar microdiscectomy. What are the specific problems in this case in relation to the pregnancy? (50%)

# Question 10

a) List the causes of reduced conscious level in a 40-year-old male presenting to the Emergency Department. (30%)
b) What do you understand by the terms primary brain injury (PBI) and secondary brain injury (SBI) as applied to traumatic brain injury (TBI)?
Outline pathophysiological mechanisms for both. (60%)

# Question 11

a) Regarding spinal anaesthesia, what factors affect the spread of injected local anaesthetic solution? (70%)
b) What symptoms and signs would you expect to see in a patient with a high spinal blockade? (20%)

## Question 12

a) What criteria would lead you to consider starting renal replacement on a patient on the intensive care unit? (20%)

b) Describe the principles behind the filtration mechanism of the continuous renal replacement device used in your intensive care unit. (40%)

c) What are the risks of continuous renal replacement on the intensive care unit? (30%)

# Paper 8

Three hour paper. Answer all the questions.
Where we have indicated the way marks are allocated, candidates are advised to spend their time accordingly.
10% of the marks for each question would be awarded for clarity, judgement and the ability to prioritise; marks would be deducted for serious errors.

## Question 1

a) Draw a diagram showing the anatomy and relationships of the epidural space at the level of the tenth and eleventh thoracic vertebrae in the transverse plane. (40%)
b) Describe how you would seek consent for thoracic epidural analgesia in a patient listed for anterior resection. (50%)

## Question 2

Outline the options for postoperative analgesia in a 71-year-old man who is undergoing pneumonectomy for adenocarcinoma of the lung. He has no other significant co-morbidities. (90%)

## Question 3

a) Outline the clotting cascade and use it to illustrate the mechanism of action of recombinant factor VIIa. (40%)
b) When might recombinant factor VIIa prove of benefit in clinical practice? (15%)
c) Explain what happens to this cascade in the development of disseminated intravascular coagulopathy (DIC). (35%)

## Question 4

a) What is the mechanism by which hypoxia can precipitate a sickle cell crisis? (30%)
b) What are the anaesthetic considerations in the perioperative period when anaesthetising a known HbSC patient undergoing elective knee replacement? (60%)

## Question 5

a) What are the specific preoperative concerns one might have in a 35-year-old lady with known systemic lupus erythematosus (SLE) who is presenting for laparoscopic cholecystectomy? (60%)
b) List the potential complications of corticosteroid treatment commonly used in patients with this condition. (30%)

## Question 6

At preassessment clinic a patient for rhinoplasty informs you that he has smoked 20 cigarettes a day for the last 20 years. He is thinking about quitting smoking. He asks whether it is a good idea to stop before the surgery or to wait until the operation is out of the way. What advice would you give him? (90%)

## Question 7

a) Define sepsis. (15%)
b) In the Surviving Sepsis Campaign, what are the key points in the resuscitation bundle (25%) and in the management bundle? (20%)
c) What is the point of providing care bundles (15%) and how have they been criticised? (15%)

## Question 8

With reference to medical statistics, define and illustrate with clinical examples the following terms:

a) Normal distribution. (20%)
b) Type I and type II error. (30%)
c) Sensitivity and specificity. (40%)

## Question 9

a) What is the definition of status epilepticus? (20%)
b) List the possible causes. (30%)
c) Outline your initial management of the convulsing patient presenting in the Emergency Department. (40%)

## Question 10

a) What is the difference between decontamination, cleaning, disinfection and sterilisation? (30%)
b) List the techniques used for sterilisation of medical equipment. (30%)
c) Describe how a reusable Classic Laryngeal Mask Airway™(LMA) is decontaminated prior to it being safe to use again. (30%)

## Question 11

a) List the contraindications to regional anaesthesia for phacoemulsification of cataract surgery. (40%)
b) What are the potential advantages of sub-Tenon's anaesthesia versus topical anaesthesia for cataract surgery? (50%)

## Question 12

a) A woman in labour has an epidural in situ. Unfortunately she is experiencing moderate (6/10) pain with contractions. This is predominantly right-sided in a T10–T12 distribution. Outline your management. (50%)
b) 6 hours later the same woman needs to go to theatre for a trial of instrumental delivery as the CTG shows late decelerations. She has received an infusion of local anaesthetic / fentanyl mix with no bolus doses within the last 2 hours. Her epidural is again patchy – what are your options? (40%)

# Paper 9

Three hour paper. Answer all the questions.
Where we have indicated the way marks are allocated, candidates are advised to spend their time accordingly.
10% of the marks for each question would be awarded for clarity, judgement and the ability to prioritise; marks would be deducted for serious errors.

## Question 1

a) What are the disadvantages of using nitrous oxide as part of a general anaesthetic for major surgery? (70%)
b) What are the benefits? (20%)

## Question 2

a) What are the factors that determine the amount of fluid moving through a tube per unit time (flow)? (50%)
b) Anaesthetists often refer to the size of medical tubes using the French or the Gauge system. What are these systems and how do they differ? (40%)

## Question 3

a) Describe a system for classifying subarachnoid haemorrhage (SAH) severity. (30%)
b) Write a checklist for the intensive care management of a patient with SAH requiring ventilation. (60%)

## Question 4

A patient 2 days post emergency laparotomy for duodenal perforation and four quadrant peritonitis is still ventilated on ITU due to evolving acute respiratory distress syndrome (ARDS). Having been in sinus rhythm at 100bpm she suddenly goes into atrial fibrillation (AF) at a rate of 160bpm.
a) What are the possible causes? (30%)
b) Outline your immediate management. (60%)

## Question 5

A 23-year-old previously fit and well motorcyclist has an acute, traumatic and appa-rently incomplete cord lesion at C7 level following a road traffic accident 4 hours previously. The surgeons need to take him to theatre for cervical spine stabilisation and also repair of a comminuted compound wrist fracture.

Outline the anaesthetic problems together with possible solutions pertinent to this case. (90%)

## Question 6

a) What is the transverse abdominal plane? Describe the afferent nerve supply blocked by deposition of local anaesthetic in this plane. (30%)
b) What are the indications for anaesthetic blockade of the transverse abdominal plane? (20%)
c) How may anaesthetic blockade of the transverse abdominal plane be performed? (40%)

## Question 7

A 71-year-old gentleman becomes steadily more confused during transurethral resection of the prostate gland (TURP) under spinal anaesthesia. You suspect TUR syndrome.
a) What is the mechanism for this condition? (30%)
b) What is the management? (30%)
c) How can the risk of developing this be reduced intraoperatively? (30%)

## Question 8

Outline
a) the potential advantages (50%) and
b) the disadvantages (40%)
of using ultrasound guidance when performing a peripheral nerve block.

## Question 9

a) What is the mechanism of action of volatile anaesthetic agents? (60%)
b) Why, when you reduce the flows in a circle system to 'ultra low flow' (<500ml/minute), do you need to increase the percentage of delivered volatile agent in order to maintain a steady volatile concentration? (30%)

## Question 10

a) How are upper gastrointestinal varices formed? (30%)
b) Describe the physical and pharmacological methods used specifically in the management of an acute variceal bleed. (40%)
c) What can be done to reduce the risk of variceal bleeds in patients known to have varices? (20%)

## Question 11

a) What are the advantages and disadvantages of pressure-control ventilation when compared to volume-control ventilation? (40%)
b) What information would lead you to believe that a patient is ready to wean from a ventilator? (50%)

# Question 12

a) How would you assess a patient's risk preoperatively of developing a venous thromboembolism (VTE)? (60%)

b) Briefly outline the non-pharmacological prophylaxis of VTE indicating with particular reference to when each modality should be used. (40%)

# Model Answers

# Paper 1

Below are the model answers for this paper. ✶✶ indicates essential information, ✶ indicates desirable information and unstarred text is supplementary information. As a guide, an answer with all the essential information and some desirable information would score 50% of the available points.

## Question 1

a)  Illustrate the anatomy of the femoral triangle and its contents. (35%)
b)  List the indications for a 'three-in-one block'. (20%)
c)  How would you perform a fascia iliaca block? (35%)

### Additional Notes

It is imperative to give a title to your diagram and label it fully. Remember to be explicit about the boundaries of the triangle as this is an important anatomical definition.

The fascia iliaca block is catching on as a useful alternative to the classic three-in-one block. It is simple to do and worth knowing for your personal practice as well as the exam.

### Answer

a) See Figure 2.

**The Femoral Triangle ★★**

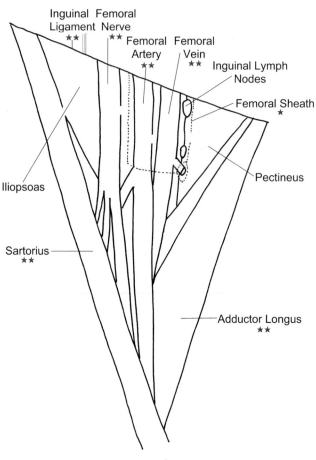

Figure 2

Boundaries

Superior – inguinal ligament
Floor – adductor longus, pectineus, iliopsoas (medial to lateral)★★
Roof – fascia lata★★
Lateral – medial border of sartorius★★
Medial – medial border of adductor longus★★

b) Block indications

Desired anaesthesia or analgesia of the following nerves:

Femoral★
Obturator★
Lateral cutaneous nerve of the thigh★

The block may be used as a sole anaesthetic:
Femoral muscle biopsy★★
Excision or suturing of lesions in the proximal anterior, lateral or medial thigh.

The block may be used as adjunctive analgesia:
Orthopaedic procedures e.g. total knee replacement, femoral neck or shaft surgery.★★
Vascular procedures such as bypass grafting.★★
Together with sciatic nerve block allowing complete analgesia of the lower limb.★★

c) Fascia iliaca block

The femoral sheath probably does not extend proximally to a sufficient distance to allow reliable spread of anaesthetic agent to the point of origin of the lateral femoral cutaneous nerve.
For this reason, a fascia iliaca block guarantees analgesia over the lateral aspect of the thigh where the 3-in-1 block may not.

Patients must be fully consented and have intravenous access in situ.★★
The block should be performed in a clean, well lit environment with resuscitation drugs and equipment and fully trained assistance available.★★
Patients should be supine.★
Sterile technique: prep and drape.★★
Locate point of needle insertion site 1cm inferior to the union of the lateral and medial two-thirds of the inguinal ligament.★★
Insert an uninsulated 20 or 22G 50mm needle perpendicular to the skin in all planes feeling for the first 'click' as the fascia lata is breached and then a second 'click' as the fascia iliaca is breached.★★
Inject 30ml of the desired local anaesthetic agent incrementally after prior aspiration.★★

The use of ultrasound may more accurately identify the fascia iliaca compartment and reduce the risk of failure or nerve damage.

### Reference
Dalens B, Vanneuville G, Tanguy A. Comparison of the fascia iliaca compartment block with the 3-in-1 block in children. *Anesth Analg* 1989; **69**: 705–13. Erratum in: *Anesth Analg* 1990; **70**: 474.

## Question 2

What are the specific problems in the anaesthetic management of a patient with acromegaly undergoing transphenoidal hypophysectomy? (90%)

### Additional Notes
Despite being an extremely rare condition (6–8 cases per 1 000 000 population) acromegaly lends itself well to a question as it is a condition that has multi-system implications. There are two ways to tackle this question. One is to take a systems approach, the other a preoperatively, intraoperatively, postoperatively one. Either works. Remember in a question like this breadth of answer will score well. A key word in the question is specific. General problems applicable to pituitary surgery – positioning, post-op endocrine abnormalities, cranial nerve dysfunction and CSF leakage – are not specific to acromegalic patients so do not form part of the answer.

### Answer
Acromegaly is caused by excess growth hormone production★★ usually by or secondary to a tumour affecting the anterior pituitary.★★

Main areas of concern are:

Cardiorespiratory★★

Cardiac disease is a major cause of morbidity and mortality in acromegalic patients.

Hypertension occurs in up to 40% of patients★ and may be resistant to treatment★ so they often present on a number of anti-hypertensives, making drug interaction more likely in this patient group.

Left ventricular hypertrophy★ occurs both in the hypertensive and normotensive acromegalic and cardiomyopathy tends to result in diastolic rather than systolic dysfunction.

Small vessel coronary artery disease has been described as has bundle branch block and approximately 50% present at surgery with ECG changes, e.g. ST depression, T wave abnormalities and conduction defects.

Airway★★

Bag/mask ventilation is straightforward in the overwhelming majority of acromegalic patients.★ However, definitive airway control may be extremely difficult.★

Acromegalic patients may have prognathism★ and macroglossia★ as well as thickening of the pharyngeal, laryngeal and vocal cords.★

Recurrent laryngeal nerve injury and laryngeal stenosis both occur and presentation with a hoarse voice should alert you to this.

Up to a quarter have an enlarged thyroid, so predisposing to sub-glottic stenosis.★ They also have an increased incidence of sleep apnoea★ (more common in male acromegalics than female; 70% vs 25%), which is predominantly secondary to upper airway obstruction but may be centrally driven.

Some patients develop a kyphosis, which can further impede easy airway manipulation.★

Endocrine★★

These patients are frequently glucose-intolerant with up to 25% being overtly diabetic.★ This may further contribute towards cardiovascular disease and may require a sliding-scale regime to be instituted in the perioperative period.

Due to local tumour effects these patients may be hypothyroid and addisonian secondary to reduced TSH and ACTH.★

Perioperative steroid replacement may be necessary.★

Raised intracranial pressure (ICP).★

Presentation can be with visual field defects which should be carefully documented preoperatively and other signs of raised ICP should be noted as well.★

Other

Unusual drugs.

Somatostatin analogues can cause vomiting and diarrhoea so check U + Es.

Bromocriptine used to lower growth hormone levels may cause severe postural hypotension.

Proximal myopathy can be severe in these patients, making mobilisation difficult. Peripheral nerve neuropraxia is more common due to soft tissue swelling so great care must be taken with padding and positioning.★

## References

Smith M, Hirsch N. Pituitary disease and anaesthesia. *Br J Anaesth* 2000; **85**: 3–14.
Nemergut E, Dumont A, Barry U, Laws E. Perioperative management of patients undergoing transphenoidal pituitary surgery. *Anesth Analg* 2005; **101**: 1170–81.

# Question 3

a) A fit 28-year-old primigravida with an uncomplicated pregnancy of 39 weeks gestation is in labour and has a cervical dilatation of 8cm. She rapidly becomes breathless and collapses with a weak pulse. What is the differential diagnosis? (30%)

b) What clinical features would suggest that the diagnosis is one of amniotic fluid embolus? (30%)

c) What would be your immediate management of this patient? (30%)

## Additional Notes

A subdivision of 'related to pregnancy' and 'unrelated to pregnancy' is always a useful starting point in a question of this nature. It should help trigger otherwise forgotten points.

Amniotic fluid embolus is a condition with which you must be familiar. Do not forget the extrathoracic considerations associated with it. Fortunately an 'ABCDE' answer is almost expected in order to show a logical approach for the last part of the question.

## Answer

a) Causes related to pregnancy:

Amniotic fluid embolus★★
Venous thromboembolism and pulmonary embolus★★
Antepartum haemorrhage (abruption or placenta praevia)★★
Pre-eclamptic pulmonary oedema★★
Peripartum cardiomyopathy★
Tocolytic pulmonary oedema (secondary to tocolytics)
Ruptured uterus

Causes unrelated to pregnancy:

Cardiac
Haemorrhage, arrhythmia, failure, myocardial infarct, valvular lesion★★
Abnormal anatomy (e.g. right to left shunt as in Eisenmenger's syndrome, previous surgery), fluid overload, septic shock★

Respiratory
Alveolar (pneumonia, ARDS, fibrosis), bronchial (asthma), upper airway (obstructive sleep apnoea, foreign body)★★

CNS
Intracerebral event, e.g. CVA★★

Drugs
Anaphylaxis, high epidural block, local anaesthetic toxicity, opiate overdose★

Blood
Transfusion error (e.g. acute haemolytic transfusion reaction, TRALI)

b) Amniotic fluid embolus (AFE) is suggested by the triad of:

Acute peripartum hypoxia★★
Coagulopathy★★
Haemodynamic collapse★★

The condition is often fatal, with survivors having significant neurological impairment. Risk factors for the development of AFE include:

Pregnancy
High maternal age, polyhydramnios, macrosomia, intrauterine death★★

Labour
    Long labour, use of oxytocics ✶
Iatrogenic
    Artificial rupture of membranes, amniocentesis or termination of pregnancy.

c)  This a life-threatening emergency – ABCDE approach ✶✶:

Call for consultant assistance ✶✶

Airway
    Assess, open and maintain the airway. Administer 100% oxygen. ✶✶

Breathing
    Examine the chest, assess the adequacy and efficacy of the respiratory effort
    (respiratory rate, $SaO_2$, ABG). ✶✶
    Support with bag-valve mask, then intubate and ventilate with cricoid pressure
    if necessary. ✶✶
    Obtund the pressor response to laryngoscopy. ✶

Circulation
    Left lateral tilt and assess pulse, BP, peripheral perfusion, heart sounds, assess
    calves for DVT. ✶✶
    12-lead ECG, continuous ECG/BP/$SaO_2$ monitoring. ✶✶
    Cannulate, take blood (send FBC, clotting, G&S, U&E, LFT, uric acid,
    magnesium). ✶✶
    Support the circulation – fluid, blood, vasopressors, ALS protocol if cardiac arrest. ✶✶
    Perimorbid caesarean section for maternal reasons if inadequate resuscitation
    within 5min.
    Look for and treat coagulopathy with FFP, platelets and cryoprecipitate. Seek
    haematological advice. ✶

Disability
    Assess neurological state – exclude intracerebral cause. ✶
    Fitting may be due to eclampsia, cerebral hypoxia or electrolyte abnormalities;
    manage all three together if uncertain aetiology. ✶

Expose
    Check for bleeding (speculum examination warranted), rashes or drug error.
    Management adjuncts include CVP, PA and peripheral arterial lines. ✶
    Investigations will include urine dipstick for proteinuria, CXR, echo, CTPA. ✶

**Reference**
Dedhia JD, Mushambi MC. Amniotic fluid embolism. *Contin Educ Anaesth Crit Care
Pain* 2007; **7**: 152–6.

## Question 4

a)  What factors increase the risk of intraoperative aspiration of abdominal contents?
    (45%)
b)  How would you reduce the risk of significant aspiration in the perioperative
    period? (45%)

**Additional Notes**
This is standard fare for an exam question and topical as there has been quite a lot in the
recent literature. The subtle change in wording for the second part of the question is
designed to test that you understand that what you aspirate may be as important as
whether you aspirate or not.

**Answer**

a) Factors increasing the risk of intraoperative aspiration:

Patient factors

Full stomach★★ / delayed gastric emptying★★

Recent meal★★

Diabetes mellitus

Raised intracranial pressure

High cord lesion

Gastrointestinal obstruction★★

Previous upper abdominal surgery

Recent trauma / severe pain★★

Recent opiate medication★

Pregnancy★

Obesity★★

Due to raised intra-abdominal pressure and increased incidence of hiatus hernia★

Known pre-existing reflux / hiatus hernia★★

Operative factors

Upper abdominal surgery★

Lithotomy position

Head-down position★

Laparoscopic surgery★

Increasing length of surgery

Anaesthetic factors

Topically anaesthetised airway.★

Insufficient depth of anaesthetic causing coughing, hiccoughs, laryngospasm or gagging.

Use of a supraglottic airway device if incorrectly seated or too high positive inspiratory pressures are used, causing gastric distension.

Use of a supraglottic airway device per se is contentious as a risk factor.

Removal of an airway device before protective reflexes are fully re-established.★★

Drugs. Opioids, atropine, glycopyrrolate, propofol, and isoflurane all decrease lower oesophageal sphincter tone.★

b) Reduction of risk in the perioperative period can be achieved by:

Avoid general anaesthesia or if required insert an appropriate airway device.★★

Control of gastric contents:

Preoperative fasting guidelines of 2 hours for clear liquids and 6 hours for solids as recommended by the American Society of Anesthesiologists (ASA) remain reasonable and adherence to these reduces the risk of pulmonary aspiration.★★

Reducing gastric acidity using $H_2$ receptor antagonists or proton pump inhibitors in high-risk patients.★ Both groups increase gastric pH and reduce gastric volumes but the number of patients needed to treat to obtain benefit for an individual is enormous. Alternatively, the buffering agent, sodium citrate, is still widely used in obstetric anaesthesia.★

Nasogastric tube (NG) insertion. Good evidence to aspirate contents of stomach if NG tube already in situ.★ Less clear whether passing an NG tube just prior to induction is of any benefit.

Avoidance, if possible, of drugs known to delay gastric emptying in the preoperative period.

Reduction in gastro-oesophageal reflux (GOR) and prevention of pulmonary aspiration:

Rapid sequence induction including cricoid pressure.★★

Care over patient positioning in known high-risk patients.★

Choice of airway device.★★ There are now a huge number of airway devices in use and there is conflicting literature as to their efficacy in preventing GOR. Endotracheal intubation remains the gold standard.★

Attenuation of the effects of aspiration:

Prompt identification is key so further aspiration is prevented★★ and the patient can be monitored in an appropriate environment postoperatively.★★ There is no evidence for either corticosteroids or prophylactic antibiotics following aspiration.

### References

Ng A, Smith G. Gastroesophageal reflux and aspiration of gastric contents in anesthetic practice. *Anesth Analg* 2001; **93**: 494–513. Online at http://www.anesthesia-analgesia. org/cgi/reprint/93/2/494. (Accessed 28 December 2008.)
Asai T. Who is at risk of pulmonary aspiration? *Br J Anaesth* 2004; **93**: 497–500.

## Question 5

An anxious 54-year-old lady requires a laparotomy for large bowel obstruction under general anaesthesia. At the preoperative visit she informs you that she is currently involved in litigation following a period of awareness under anaesthesia for haemorrhoidectomy.

Summarise the points you would raise in the preoperative discussion in relation to awareness and her proposed anaesthetic. (90%)

### Additional Notes

This question seeks out those candidates who have progressed beyond the standard of a year 1 or 2 anaesthetic trainee in terms of clinical maturity, patient communication skills and theoretical knowledge. Try to show in your discussion with the patient that you know why awareness may occur and how to prevent it.

Think more of what you would do if you were placed in this situation rather than worrying about what the examiners are after.

### Answer

Delicate situation; consider discussion with a senior anaesthetist.★★

Two aspects in providing good care and avoiding further litigation:

1. Acquisition of the details of the aforementioned operation.

Collection of notes and legal documentation.★★

Interview the patient to obtain her version of events.★★

Ascertain:

Emergency or elective operation?★★

Type of anaesthesia used and in what dose?★★

Airway difficulty (increased chance of awareness)?★

Discern whether true intraoperative awareness – recall of conversation, sensation of pain, do descriptions tie in with the anaesthetic/surgical events or do events appear to be recovery-room-based or recall from a period of ventilation on the ICU?★★

If true awareness, has she had a formal debrief? How has it affected her – insomnia, depression, post-traumatic stress disorder?★★

2. Minimisation of (a) awareness and (b) litigation in this case.

a) Explain the steps that you will take to minimise awareness:

Identify and/or treat problem which raises MAC, e.g. hyperthyroidism, excessive alcohol/recreational drug use (e.g. cocaine). ✷

Thorough machine and equipment check. ✷

Use benzodiazepine, e.g. midazolam 5mg on induction. ✷✷

Consider clonidine to reduce MAC. ✷

Volatile agent anaesthesia facilitating end-tidal agent monitoring (minimises variability in minimum inhibitory concentration seen with IV anaesthesia). ✷✷

Maintenance of >1 MAC with use of vasopressors to support BP if needed. ✷✷

Concomitant regional technique, e.g. epidural or TAP block to reduce MAC.

Multimodal analgesia

Use of a technique to detect awareness and therefore act on it (e.g. BIS monitor) is controversial. ✷✷

b) Minimise the chance of litigation by ensuring:

She understands:

Surgery is essential.

All feasible measures will be taken to reduce the risk of awareness, e.g. the 'safety' of not using neuromuscular blockers may be enhanced by use of remi-fentanil. ✷

Consultant anaesthetist overseeing care. ✷✷

Despite this, another episode of awareness may occur. ✷✷

Include this on the consent form and ensure it is signed. ✷✷

Keep meticulous notes of preoperative discussion, drugs administered, regular end-tidal measurements, physiological values and the results of regular intraoperative patient examination. ✷✷

### Reference

Hardman JG, Aitkenhead AR. Awareness during anaesthesia. *Contin Educ Anaesth Crit Care Pain* 2005; **5**: 183–6.

## Question 6

a) List the complications of blood transfusion that may occur within the operating theatre. (50%)

b) Outline the steps that need to be taken to ensure a unit of packed red cells received by the patient is the correct one. (40%)

### Additional Notes

The first part is a classic classify-or-die answer. Remember to read the question carefully. No marks will be awarded for late complications. It's good to think of your answer in terms of the potential complications of giving one drop of blood and the complications of giving lots (i.e. multiple units) of blood products. Remember the following reactions can occur from administration of all types of blood product (FFP, packed red cells, platelets, etc.). Though incorrect/incompatible blood product administration causes the most serious immunological complications, they do occur with 'correct' product administration.

The second part is a 'close your eyes and imagine you are there' type scenario. Writing down what you have done many times in your career already can be harder than you think! The AAGBI have recently published on this and the SHOT study website is informative reading (references below).

## Answer

a) Complications of transfusion can be classified into three main groups.

Immunological★★

Leukocyte-depleted blood★ was introduced in the UK in 1998. This was initiated due to the perceived benefit of a reduction in Creutzfeldt-Jakob disease (vCJD) transmission and immunosuppression. The incidence of immunological complications has reduced considerably. Immunological complications can be divided into those associated with incorrect component administration,★★ e.g. ABO incompatibility, and those without.★★

Haemolytic reactions (can be acute or delayed).

Former due usually to ABO incompatibility.★ Presents with hypotension, rash, reduced lung compliance, pulmonary oedema and tachycardia.★★ Treat as for anaphylactic reaction.★★

Acute transfusion reactions.

Often due to minor antigen/antibody incompatibility. Vary from isolated febrile reaction to fever with hypotension to minor allergy (e.g. skin rash) through to severe anaphylactic/anaphylactoid reaction and ARDS.★★

Infective★★

Viral★: HIV, hepatitis, cytomegalovirus, human T-cell leukaemia and lymphoma virus type 1 (HTLV-I)

Bacteria★: usually due to bag contamination.

Other: malaria, prion disease★.

Other including metabolic★

(Tend to be associated more with large-volume blood transfusion).

Hyperkalaemia★★

Hypocalcaemia★

Coagulopathy due to coagulation factor depletion★★

Impaired oxygen delivery due to left shift of oxyhaemoglobin dissociation curve★

Hypothermia★★

Fluid overload (pulmonary oedema, hypertension)★

Complications involved in the actual administration process such as air embolism, problems of intravenous access

b) To ensure the patient receives the correct blood:

Two pairs of eyes are better than one. Do not cut corners even in the most life-threatening haemorrhage.★★

Make sure the theatre personnel fetching the blood take a slip containing adequate patient information to minimise the chance of the wrong blood being brought.★★

Confirm the identity of the patient.★★ Look at the patient,★ their name band★★ and notes if possible. A patient name band should be attached to the patient.★★

Cross-check the blood compatibility label on the bag with the paper slip that comes with the blood.★★ This must correspond with the patient.★★ This includes name,★★ date of birth,★★ hospital number,★★ ABO status,★ rhesus status, expiry date.★

Confirm the integrity of the blood bag's plastic casing.★

Record that the blood has been administered★★ (usually a peel-off sticky label) and keep the blood bag for later identification should a problem arise.★

## References

SHOT Survey. Online at www.shotuk.org. (Accessed 28 December 2008.)

AAGBI Guideline. Blood Transfusion and the Anaesthetist. June 2008; 2nd edn. Online at www.aagbi.org/publications/guidelines/docs/red_cell_08.pdf. (Accessed 28 December 2008.)

# Question 7

a) How do you select an appropriately sized blood pressure cuff for a patient? (10%)
b) What are the principles behind the non-invasive methods of blood pressure measurement? (40%)
c) The measurement of invasive blood pressure requires a transducer. What is a transducer and what is its mechanism of action in this context? (40%)

## Additional Notes

A question on the physics of blood pressure measurement was asked in May 2006. It was answered extremely poorly and exactly the same question was asked again in May 2007. It was again answered very poorly but has not been asked a third time. Understanding the principles behind the measurement of blood pressure is a core skill in anaesthesia and so it would not be unreasonable to expect a similar question to be asked once more.

## Answer

a) The cuff should have a width of 40% of the mid-arm circumference, or be 20% wider than the arm's diameter. ★★
   It should cover 2/3 of the length of the arm. ★★
   The centre of the bladder should lie over the medial side of the arm. ★

b) Manual
   The artery is occluded with a pneumatic cuff, the pressure in which is measured by a bourdon or anaeroid gauge. ★★
   On cuff deflation, a point is reached at which the systolic pressure is high enough to force blood beneath the cuff, causing turbulent flow of blood in the artery, stretching and reverberation of the vessel. These phenomena are detectable with an ultrasound device (e.g. doppler), stethoscope (first Korotkoff sound) or by palpation. ★★
   At the diastolic pressure, arterial constriction ends, blood flow becomes laminar, reverberation of the vessel wall ceases and the fifth Korotkoff sound is heard. ★★

   Automated methods, e.g. DINAMAP (device for non-invasive automatic mean arterial pressure).
   These systems utilise the principle of oscillometry and are based on the workings of the Von Recklinghausen oscillotonometer. ★★
   The systolic pressure is identified by the point at which a sensing needle first oscillates as the cuff is deflated from a point above systolic pressure. ★★
   The oscillations then reduce in amplitude before increasing to maximal at the mean arterial pressure. ★★
   The diastolic pressure is then calculated although some devices may measure it as a secondary feature, being the point of maximal rate of oscillation decrease. ★★

c) A transducer is a device which converts one form of energy into another. ★
   In the case of invasive arterial pressure measurement, the transducer converts the kinetic energy of a column of pressurised fluid into electrical energy for display on the monitoring device. ★★
   The motion of blood in the vessel drives the column of fluid as the two are hydraulically coupled via the arterial cannula. ★
   This results in movement of the diaphragm and in turn the strain gauge (Figure 3), the resistance of which increases with increasing length. ★★
   When incorporated into a Wheatstone bridge the current produced is proportional to the initial diaphragmatic displacement and therefore the blood pressure. ★★
   The varying current is then displayed electronically as the arterial waveform.

**Schematic View of Arterial Pressure Transducer** ★ ★

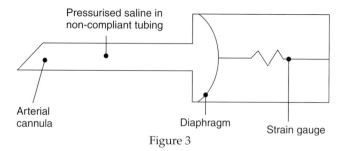

Figure 3

### References

Davis PD, Kenny GNC. Electricity. In: *Basic physics and measurement in anaesthesia*, 5th edition. Butterworth Heinemann. 2005; 161–2.
Ward M, Langton JA. Blood pressure measurement. *Contin Educ Anaesth Crit Care Pain* 2007; 7: 122–6.

## Question 8

A 46-year-old 95kg previously healthy patient is brought into the emergency department having been extricated from a burning car by the fire brigade following a motor vehicle collision. He has burns to the face and significant circumferential burns to the torso and upper limbs and the GCS was recorded as 13.

a) What in particular would you be looking for during your initial survey of this patient? (35%)
b) What intraoperative problems might you predict were this patient to be taken to theatre for debridement of his burns? (40%)
c) List the drugs you would have drawn up at induction, 3 hours after the vehicle accident, giving the doses you would expect to administer. (15%)

### Additional Notes

Reasonable 'burns' questions which may be asked concern the practical aspects of anaesthetic care both immediately and in the days or weeks subsequent to the initial event, fluid management and pharmacological changes subsequent to burns. A basic knowledge of burn pathophysiology is also required.
This question ties in several of these topics and will require you to think laterally as well as think ahead; a realistic expectation!
Look carefully for key words in the question: '… circumferential burns… ', 'what in particular…' all guide you to the information the examiner is looking for.

### Answer

a) Pathology relating to:
   Burns
   Trauma
   Medical problems coexisting/responsible for the collision.

Airway and C-spine
   Airway burn (nasal hair singeing, airway soot, carbonaceous sputum, stridor/wheeze, erythema and swelling). ★ ★

Anatomical distortion making early intubation difficult (airway oedema is likely to worsen dramatically).✶✶
Ensure hard collar/blocks/tape and spinal immobilisation.✶✶

Breathing
Circumferential burns to the torso raise likelihood of respiratory failure, which would warrant escharotomies (do serial ABGs).✶✶
Smoke inhalation may result in acute lung injury (do CXR).✶
Carbon monoxide/cyanide poisoning may produce histotoxic hypoxia and low GCS.✶✶
Carboxyhaemoglobin – spuriously high $SpO_2$ readings (measure COHb).✶
Chest trauma, e.g. fractures, pneumo/haemothoraces.✶✶
The patient's size may further embarrass the breathing.

Circulation
Identify and stop bleeding/shock from additional injuries (chest/abdominal/pelvic/long bone examination $\pm$ CXR/Focussed assessment with sonography for trauma (FAST)/CT).✶✶
Estimate additional fluid requirements (Parkland formula).✶✶
Assess neurovascular supply to the upper limbs (circumferential burns may warrant escharotomies to maintain perfusion).✶✶
Exclude cardiac event causing or stemming from trauma (do ECG).

Disability
GCS 13 raises chance of head injury. CT head mandatory.✶✶
Improper spinal immobilisation may have resulted during extrication from burning vehicle; assess neurology carefully prior to intubation.

Expose
Further burns/trauma. Estimate burn area.✶✶
Catheterise – guide resuscitation/myoglobinuria?✶
Keep warm.✶✶
Remove jewellery.

b) Problems:
Airway
Accidental extubation disastrous as airway may be swollen.

Breathing
High minute volumes required given a hypermetabolic state.✶
Airway burn increases physiological dead space – $ETCO_2$ not reflective of $PaCO_2$.✶

Circulation
Skin loss predisposes to large fluid losses – CVP line needed.✶✶
Wide-bore IV access difficult given burned skin.✶✶
Circumferential limb burn impedes proximal passage of fluid.✶✶
Excessive blood loss and massive transfusion – 1% BSA excised loses 3–4% of the circulating volume.✶✶
Coagulopathy can easily develop.✶✶
Alteration in $V_d$ of drugs requiring dose adjustment.

Anaesthesia
Burns theatre may be isolated.✶
Difficulties monitoring, e.g. placing ECG electrodes.✶✶
Prolonged operation – patient positioning.✶✶

High analgesic requirements.

Hypothermia with associated depression in cardiovascular, respiratory, metabolic and haemostatic function.★★ Forced air warming inefficient due to patient exposure. Warm theatre essential (30°C).★★

Prone to infection; care with asepsis.★

Rhabdomyolysis and associated complications, e.g. hyperkalaemia, renal failure. Hypermetabolic and catabolic.

c) Drugs
   Thiopentone 175mg★★
   Suxamethonium 150mg★★
   Alfentanil 2000µg★★
   Metaraminol 0.5–1mg
   Ephedrine 3–6mg
   Atropine 300mcg
   Spare suxamethonium150mg
   Atracurium 50mg
   Naloxone 400mcg

**Reference**

Black RG, Kinsella J. Anaesthetic management for burns patients. *Contin Educ Anaesth Crit Care Pain* 2001; **6**: 177–80.

# Question 9

a) What is your choice of crystalloid for intravenous intraoperative fluid replacement in paediatric anaesthesia? Outline why some fluids are less suitable than your first choice. (50%)
b) How would you calculate the maintenance fluid regimen for a child? (20%)
c) Why might you fluid-restrict a sick child? (20%)

**Answer**

a) Intravenous fluid is advisable as it replaces deficit/ongoing loss and reduces PONV.★

Currently would choose Hartmann's solution.★★

Ideally would like a Hartmann's solution with 1% glucose but this is currently not available in our Trust.★ I would therefore monitor the blood glucose during the case and give additional glucose infusion if required.★

Fifty case reports in children of serious morbidity or death from iatrogenic hyponatremia. Usually given large volumes of hypotonic fluid on the back of already low plasma sodium.★

Dextrose 4%/saline 0.19% or dextrose 2.5%/saline 0.45% are isotonic at administration, but hypotonic when dextrose is metabolised.★★ Their administration can lead to hyponatremia.★★

All replacement fluids should be isotonic.★★

Hyponatremic children should receive isotonic fluids.★

Healthy infants maintain blood glucose during surgery with or without added dextrose.★

Concerns with hypernatremia when administering 0.9% saline/5% dextrose.★ Concerns about chloride load and acidemia. Only 1% glucose required to prevent hypoglycemia and ketosis.★ The 5% dextrose part may cause hyperglycemia. This is a hyperosmolar solution requiring more cannulas and/or central access.

b) Calculating paediatric maintenance regimen

Eighty per cent of British anaesthetists who regularly anaesthetise children use the Holliday and Segar formula ★★:

| Body weight (kg) | Average maintenance allowance for fluid | |
| --- | --- | --- |
| | ml/day | ml/hr |
| 0–10 | 100ml/kg | 4ml/kg |
| 10–20 | 1000ml + 50ml/kg for each kg more than 10kg | 40ml + 2ml/kg for each kg more than 10kg |
| 20+ | 1500ml + 20ml/kg for each kg more than 20kg | 60ml + 1ml/kg for each kg more than 20kg |

Other formulae are available. ★

c) Fluid restriction is often beneficial in sick children. ★

During acute illness factors such as stress, ★ pyrexia, ★ pain ★ and nausea ★ lead to an increase in antidiuretic hormone secretion. ★★

This is independent of osmolar effects ★ and leads to a decrease in the kidney's ability to excrete free water. ★★

The Holliday and Segar formula is designed to produce the correct fluid replacement in healthy children, not the correct tonicity in sick children. ★★

Recent reports recommend fluid-restricting sick children to 2/3 the calculated volume and regularly monitoring their electrolytes to guide fluid management. ★

### References

NPSA Recommendations. Online at http://www.npsa.nhs.uk/nrls/alerts-and-directives/alerts/intravenous-infusions/ (Accessed 1 January 2009.)

Way C, Dhamrait R, Wade A, Walker I. Perioperative fluid therapy in children: a survey of current prescribing practice. *BJA* 2006; **97**(3): 371–9.

## Question 10

Define the following:
a) Nociception (10%)
b) Allodynia (10%)
c) Hyperalgesia (10%)
d) Neuropathic pain (10%)
e) What is the mechanism of action of gabapentin and when might it be useful in the management of chronic pain? (50%)

### Additional Notes

Definitions – you either know them or you don't! Again, a trawl of the A to Z is worth it to make sure you have the common ones off pat. In well-circumscribed areas such as chronic pain there will inevitably be some repetition in question material so a look at the past pain questions is time well spent. Gabapentin is adopting a magnesium-type role in anaesthetic practice (i.e. you seem to be able to use it for just about anything) so is a 'hot topic'.

### Answer

a) Nociception is not the same as pain. ★ The former is the sensation of noxious stimuli, ★★ the latter describes both an unpleasant sensory and emotional experience. Both can be associated with either actual or potential tissue damage. ★

b) Allodynia is a painful response to a usually non-painful stimulus.✳✳ It is a clinical feature of many painful conditions such as neuropathies, post-herpetic neuralgia and fibromyalgia.

c) Hyperalgesia is increased pain from a normally painful stimulus.✳✳ Tends to be a feature of chronic pain conditions. Similar to antalgesia which is increased sensitivity to painful stimuli caused by small doses of CNS depressant drugs, e.g. thiopentone.

d) Neuropathic pain is pain initiated or caused by a primary lesion or dysfunction in the nervous system.✳✳ Commonly seen in diabetic neuropathy and post-herpetic infection.

e) The mechanism of action of gabapentin is complicated. Although structurally related to GABA (gamma-aminobutyric acid) it does not interact with GABA receptors. Its main action seems to be on the alpha-2-delta subunit✳ of voltage-gated calcium channels✳✳ where it inhibits their action.✳✳ It may also:

   Stimulate glutamate decarboxylase, so increasing GABA conversion from glutamate.✳

   Increase the synaptic release of GABA (GABA is an inhibitory neurotransmitter).✳

   Antagonise action at NMDA receptors (similar to the action of drugs such as ketamine, methadone and tramadol).✳

   Have a direct effect on cell membranes.✳

Anticonvulsants, in combination with antidepressants, have been prescribed for the treatment of neuropathic pain for many years.✳ Gabapentin is currently licensed for the treatment of neuropathic pain.✳✳ A Cochrane review showed that the numbers needed to treat for an improvement in the symptoms of neuropathic pain in all patients treated with Gabapentin was 4.3 (95% CI 3.5–5.7)✳ and it had a favourable side-effect profile.✳✳ Of interest, the review also stated that there was insufficient evidence for its use in the treatment of acute pain even though there has been recent work suggesting it may be of use as an opioid-sparing agent in the perioperative period.

Gabapentin has also been used successfully in the treatment of:
Complex regional pain syndrome✳✳
The pain associated with spinal cord injury✳
Fibromyalgia pain
Migraine
Pain and spasticity seen in multiple sclerosis

### References

The International Association for the Study of Pain website is a useful resource. www.iasp-pain.org. (Accessed 30 December 2008.)

Bennett M, Simpson K. Gabapentin in the treatment of neuropathic pain. *Palliat Med* 2004; **18**: 5–11.

Gabapentin for acute and chronic pain. A Cochrane review, 20 July 2005. Online at www.cochrane.org/reviews/en/ab005452.html (Accessed 1 January 2009.)

## Question 11

Three weeks prior to admission for laparoscopic right hemicolectomy for carcinoma a 77-year-old patient attends a pre-assessment clinic. He has ischaemic heart disease, heart failure, smokes and gets short of breath after walking 50 metres on flat, level ground.

a) List the advantages of seeing this gentleman 6 weeks prior to surgery. (30%)
b) At this appointment and from subsequent investigations how could he be assessed and then, up to the day before admission, optimised for surgery? (60%)

## Additional Notes

If there is one topic that you should have a feel for this is it. There are pre-assessment clinics springing up all over the place and the College has not asked a question – yet.

Having an idea about CPEX (cardiopulmonary exercise testing) is essential. This is a big, open-ended question so make sure you plan, plan, plan! There is a clear time limit to the preoptimisation of this patient as his operation is for cancer. Remember there is still loads of optimisation that can be done in the immediate perioperative period but that's for another question....

## Answer

a) The aim of preoperative assessment is to improve outcome✷ and efficiency✷ of service. It can help do this by:

Identifying potential anaesthetic difficulties✷✷

Identifying existing medical conditions✷✷

Allowing an accurate quantification of risk which can then be discussed with the patient so allowing more informed consent✷

Providing an opportunity for explanation and discussion✷

Reducing the risk of day of surgery cancellation✷

Allowing an opportunity to optimise the patient's condition prior to surgery✷✷

All of these actions would be advantageous in this case.

b) Assessment of this patient begins with a thorough history and clinical examination.✷✷ This would ideally be done by the anaesthetist allocated to the theatre list in 6 weeks time.

An overall assessment of functional capacity can be made by assessing his MET (metabolic equivalent) capacity.✷ <4 METs and he falls into a high-risk group (unable to undertake exercise requiring a 4 × increase in resting metabolic rate such as climbing stairs).

The history and examination should be focused on, but not solely limited to, his cardiorespiratory status.✷✷ In particular, one should question whether there has been any recent worsening of functional status and if so, why.✷

He should be optimised from a coronary heart disease point of view to Canadian Class I or II angina (no worse than angina brought on by day-to-day activity but only slightly functionally limiting) and consideration may be given to anigioplastic intervention if symptoms warrant.✷

His heart failure should also be optimised medically to NYHA class I or II, if possible (no or slight limitation to physical activity).✷ An echocardiogram and ECG would both be helpful.✷

Bloods should be sent and abnormal results investigated.✷

Anaemia is common in this group so dependent on results iron supplementation / transfusion may be necessary.✷

All other routine bloods should be screened, including liver function tests, clotting studies and U + Es.✷

A blood gas on air may be of prognostic significance and give a useful 'baseline'. His drug chart should be reviewed and the patient informed of the drugs which should be continued or altered in the immediate perioperative period.✷

CPEX (cardiopulmonary exercise testing) would be extremely useful in this situation.✷ Measurement of anaerobic threshold is of prognostic significance and allows appropriate resources to be allocated at the time of admission and postoperatively.

A chest X-ray or respiratory function tests will probably add little to the above but should be ordered if specific clinical concerns arise at pre-assessment.✷

The patient should be counselled to stop smoking✷✷ and take regular exercise.

## References

Fleisher L, Beckman J, Brown K, et al. ACC/AHA guidelines on perioperative cardiovascular evaluation for non-cardiac surgery. *Circulation* 2007; **116**: e418–e500. Online at http://circ.ahajournals.org/cgi/reprint/116/17/e418 (Accessed on 1 January 2009.)
García-Miguel F, Serrano-Aguilar P, López-Bastida J. Preoperative assessment. *The Lancet* Nov 2003; **362** (9397):1749–57.

## Question 12

a) What are the indications for commencing total parenteral nutrition in a ventilated patient on intensive care? (20%)
b) How would you determine a patient's daily calorie requirement? (20%)
c) Outline the uses of lipid emulsion in anaesthesia and critical care. (50%)

### Additional Notes

The marks weighting is heavily biased towards the last section. This should draw the candidate into realising that this is the main deal. A good candidate would mention TPN (total parenteral nutrition), propofol and LA toxicity. This is specifically not made overt in the question. There is a lot to this question. This answer contains an excess of information as there are potentially many interesting points to cover. Look at the essential and desirable areas to work out how you would pare your answer into a 15-minute essay.

### Answer

a) Patients need energy to heal.
  Ideally, enterally feed patient in ITU whenever possible.✶✶
  When adequate energy cannot be supplied enterally, TPN is indicated
    to either fully feed a patient or✶
    to supplement enteral feeding.✶

  This could be because of
    impaired bowel function (e.g. prolonged ileus)✶
    impaired access to the bowel (e.g. upper gastrointestinal obstruction with failure to secure a jejunostomy).✶

  Poorly nourished patients will reduce one's threshold for commencing TPN.
  Decision should not be taken lightly as the complications of TPN may be life-threatening.✶✶

b) There are many predictive equations✶✶ for baseline calculation in health:
  Harris-Benedict equation
  Adjusted Harris-Benedict equation
  Mifflin
  Owen
  WHO

  Most factor in gender, age, height and weight.✶
  The Harris-Benedict formula dates back to 1919 and, with today's level of obesity and lack of exercise, tends to overestimate calorie requirements. The adjusted version calculates a reduced body weight in obese patients.
  The Mifflin formula adds in a factor for level of exercise.
  Maintenance for standard males is in the region of 75–90kJ/kg body weight.✶
  Often a number of formulae are used and the results averaged.
  Once a 'maintenance in health' figure is calculated, the sum is usually weighted by a factor ranging from 1.0 to 1.5.✶✶

This is affected by:
  Surgery
  Infection
  Burns
  Organ failure
  Trauma
  Cancer
  Starvation

Predictive formulae have been shown to be least accurate for obese ventilator-dependent patients.

Indirect calorimetry is the gold standard but is rarely available.✶

Metabolic monitors continuously measure oxygen consumption and carbon dioxide production, allowing determination of caloric needs and substrate utilisation.

The units are expensive and do not perform much more accurately than predictive equations.

Some models are inaccurate with $FiO_2$ above 0.6.

c) Total parenteral nutrition.✶✶

Lipid emulsion acts as:
  a source of energy for TPN✶✶
  a source of essential fatty acids✶

Being made of fat, lipid emulsion allows a high amount of energy to be infused in a small volume.✶

Fat emulsions can be used to supply up to 40% of the non-protein calorie requirements for a patient.

Each ml of 20% Intralipid contains 8.4kJ.

Care must be taken when using lipid emulsions in the presence of disorders of lipid metabolism✶ such as pancreatitis.

Local anaesthetic (LA) toxicity.✶✶

Intralipid has been shown to reverse LA-induced cardiac arrest in animal models and human case reports.✶

AAGBI guidelines March 2007.

In the presence of seizures or cardiovascular collapse following or during administration of local anaesthetic, commence CPR if indicated.

If patient not responsive, give an intravenous bolus of Intralipid 20% 1.5ml/kg over 1 minute (usually about 100ml).✶

Start an infusion of 20% Intralipid at 0.25ml/kg per min.✶

Repeat the bolus twice at 5-minute intervals if adequate circulation has not been restored.

Increase the infusion rate to 0.5ml/kg per min if adequate circulation has not been restored.

Continue infusion until an adequate circulation has been restored.

Continue CPR throughout the infusion.

Recovery from LA toxicity may take >1hr.

Propofol is not a suitable substitute for Intralipid.

Take blood samples in a plain and a heparinised tube before and after administration of lipid and at 1hr and ask lab to measure LA and triglyceride levels.

Drug presentation✶

Lipid emulsion has been used to allow injection of agents with low water solubility.✶

Over the years this has included althesin and etomidate, but its current most popular use is in the presentation of propofol.✶

Initially propofol was developed in Cremophor EL but this was withdrawn following a number of anaphylactic reactions.

Diprivan propofol is presented in
   10% soybean oil
   1.2% purified egg phospholipid (emulsifier)
   2.25% of glycerol as a tonicity adjusting agent
   and sodium hydroxide to adjust the pH.
The nutrient qualities of fat emulsion mean that they must contain an antimicrobial agent.
Diprivan contains EDTA.
The non-lipid-bound fraction of propofol is thought to be responsible for pain on injection and a new emulsion with added medium-chain triglycerides is being investigated to produce a more comfortable induction.

### References

AAGBI. Guidelines for the management of severe local anaesthetic toxicity. 2007. Online at http://www.aagbi.org/publications/guidelines/docs/latoxicity07.pdf (Accessed 30 December 2008.)

Lipid Rescue website at http://www.lipidrescue.org/ (Accessed 30 December 2008.)

# Paper 2

Below are the model answers for this paper. ⋆⋆ indicates essential information, ⋆ indicates desirable information and unstarred text is supplementary information. As a guide, an answer with all the essential information and some desirable information would score 50% of the available points.

## Question 1

a) Draw a transverse section through the axilla at the level of the inferior border of the pectoralis major at its humeral insertion, detailing the anatomical relations of the axillary artery and the brachial plexus. (50%)
b) List the surgical indications for supraclavicular blockade of the brachial plexus. (10%)
c) List the potential complications of an interscalene block. (30%)

### Additional Notes
Be sure to read the question carefully; this question examines your knowledge of three different types of approach to the brachial plexus.

The first part may seem daunting, but it merely refers to the point of needle insertion for an axillary plexus block. (As a general rule it is always worth having in your head a cross or transverse section of every anatomical site into which you may insert a needle.) Always label your drawing and orientate the figure (i.e. medial/lateral) as failure to do so may score few marks.

## Answer

a) See Figure 4.

**Transverse Section Through the Axilla at the Humeral Insertion of Pectoralis Major ★ ★**

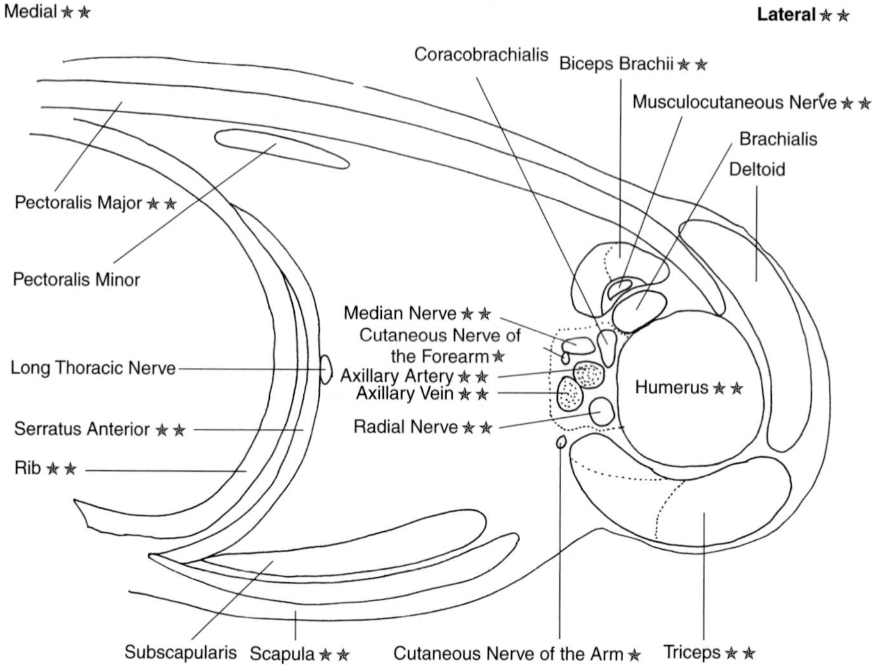

Figure 4

b) Supraclavicular blockade is most suited to surgery involving the elbow, forearm or hand. ★★

c) Complications include:

Those secondary to needling:

Bleeding (vascular injury to subclavian artery, vertebral artery, internal or external jugular veins). ★★

Nerve injury (intraneural needle placement). May affect brachial plexus ★★ or other nerves in the proximity, e.g. ansa cervicalis, ★ phrenic, ★ vagus ★ or recurrent laryngeal nerves. ★

Pneumothorax ★★

Infection ★★

Those secondary to local anaesthetic:

Intravascular injection – CNS and CVS toxicity with cardiovascular collapse. ★★

Intraneural injection with nerve injury (see above). ★★

Anaesthetising the phrenic nerve will result in impaired respiratory function and anaesthetising the sympathetic chain will result in Horner syndrome. ★

Total spinal or epidural spread of anaesthetic. ★★

Local anaesthetic toxicity. ★★

Allergic reactions. ★

## References

Moore KL, Dalley AF. The upper limb. In: *Clinically orientated anatomy*, 4th edition. Lippincott Williams & Wilkins. 1999; 694–716.

The New York Society of Regional Anaesthesia website. http://nysora.com/techniques/ (Accessed 30 September 2008.)

# Question 2

a) Briefly outline the treatment options for weight reduction available to a patient with Class III obesity (BMI >40). (60%)

b) When anaesthetising this patient, how would you optimise oxygenation and position the patient for intubation prior to induction? (30%)

## Additional Notes

Obesity is common and on the increase. Add to this the recent NICE Guidelines on many aspects of obesity and it becomes a topic area that the College visits regularly.

## Answer

a) Weight reduction may be achieved through:

Diet,✶✶ exercise✶✶ and behavioural therapy✶ with a particular focus on energy imbalance (calories eaten versus calories expended).✶

Drug treatment
This is indicated when BMI>27 with co-morbidities✶ or >30 without.✶
Two groups – appetite suppressants and those that decrease absorption.
Appetite suppressants.✶ Sibutramine✶ is a norepinephrine and serotonin reuptake inhibitor enhancing satiety and increasing BMR. May increase BP and HR, produce dry mouth, headache, nausea, insomnia and constipation.
Decreasing nutrient absorption.✶ Orlistat✶ binds to gastrointestinal lipases in the gut, preventing fat hydrolysis. Initial side effects are flatulence, steatorrhea and incontinence. Decreases ADEK absorption.

Bariatric surgery is the only treatment that can produce long-term weight reduction.✶✶ Patients usually have co-morbidity. Indicated when BMI>40✶ or >35 with co-morbidity✶ or when medical therapy has failed.✶ Gives 50% decrease in excess body weight at 18 months. Either restrict food intake (gastric banding)✶ or produce malabsorption (Roux-en-Y bypass).✶ Increasingly performed laparoscopically✶ with less pain, fewer incisional hernias and adhesions and shorter stay. During weight loss may be at risk of cholelithiasis (give ursodiol). Banding procedures are simple and initially effective but may produce reflux oesophagitis and long-term weight gain. Bypass procedures produce less initial weight loss (35%) but are more effective long-term.✶ They may produce anastamotic stenosis, Fe, B12 or ADEK deficiency, nausea and vomiting and dumping syndrome.

b) The patient should be pre-oxygenated to optimise oxygenation prior to induction.✶✶ This should be done with the patient in a 25° head-up position.✶ In a recent prospective randomised controlled trial, this position was shown to delay desaturation down to a $SaO_2$ of 92% by 46 seconds, giving a greater safety margin in Class III obese patients. This ties in well with the practice of 'ramping up' the patient for best position for laryngoscopy.✶ In this practice, the patient is positioned on a ramp of pillows or a purpose-made wedge to ensure that the head and shoulders are significantly above the chest. It has been recommended that the external auditory meatus should be at or above the level of the sternal notch.

## References

Cheah M, Kam P. Obesity: Basic science and medical aspects relevant to anaesthetists. *Anaesthesia* 2005; **60**: 1009–21.

Dixon BJ, Dixon JB, Carden JR, et al. Preoxygenation is more effective in the 25° head-up position than in the supine position in severely obese patients. *Anesthesiology* 2005; **102**: 1110–5.

NICE Guideline CG43 Online at http://www.nice.org.uk/Guidance/CG43 (Accessed 1 January 2009.)

# Question 3

a) Draw a labelled schematic diagram of a co-axial Mapleson D anaesthetic breathing system showing fresh gas flow entering the system. (30%)
b) Why is a Mapleson D inefficient for spontaneous ventilation yet efficient for intermittent positive pressure ventilation (IPPV)? (30%)
c) Give two advantages and disadvantages of a co-axial D over an unmodified system. (10%)
d) Give two ways that one can check that the inner lumen of a coaxial D (Bain) is safe to use. (20%)

## Additional Notes

There is quite a lot in this question. You should be able to draw, label and talk about all the main anaesthetic breathing systems without any difficulty. Part (b) seems to stump a lot of candidates in mock vivas.

## Answer

a) See Figure 5.

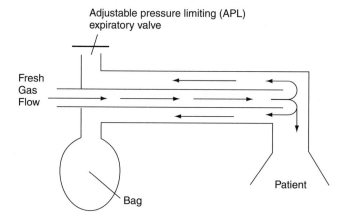

Adjustable pressure limiting (APL) expiratory valve

Fresh Gas Flow

Bag

Patient

Co-axial Mapleson D Anaesthetic Breathing System
Figure 5

Correct title★★
Co-axial system★★
Adjustable pressure-limiting (APL) expiratory valve★★
Bag★★
Patient end indicated★★
Fresh gas flow indicated★★
Inner tube ending before reaching patient★★

b) Anaesthetic breathing system efficiency is all down to what happens to the dead-space gas and whether it can be reused or not.★★ The difference between a system used for spontaneous ventilation or IPPV is whether the expiratory valve is open (as in spontaneous ventilation) or partially closed (as in IPPV).★★

Spontaneous ventilation:
In exhalation during spontaneous ventilation exhaled gas and fresh gas mix in the expiratory limb★ and travel towards the reservoir bag preceded by the dead-space gas,★ part of which will leave the circuit via the expiratory valve.★ When the bag is full the pressure in the system rises so a mixture of fresh gas and exhaled gas is vented out.★ During the expiratory pause, fresh gas flow

continues to push exhaled gas down the expiratory limb✻ but unless the fresh gas flow (FGF) is at least twice the minute volume the patient will still rebreathe some of the exhaled gas,✻ hence the system is inefficient.

IPPV:
The difference here is that the expiratory valve is partially occluded.✻✻ Hence the dead-space gas fills the bag and it is only a mixture of exhaled gas and fresh gas flow that leaves via the expiratory valve.✻ When the bag is squeezed the patient receives a mixture of fresh gas and gas that is in the bag, which is where the dead-space gas has gone.✻ Therefore rebreathing is reduced✻ hence the system is much more efficient.

c) Advantages:
Decreases the bulk of the circuit.✻✻
Retention of heat and humidity is improved as a result of partial warming of the inspiratory gases by countercurrent exchange with the warmer expired gases.✻

Disadvantages:
Cost
Disconnection or kinking of the inner tube may go unnoticed.✻✻

d) There are two ways to check whether the inner lumen (i.e. the lumen for the fresh gas flow) is patent:

The Pethick test✻
Close the expiratory valve and allow the bag to fill.✻ Once full activate the oxygen quick flush.✻ If the inner tube is intact then the rapid movement of gas down it empties the bag via a Venturi effect.✻✻ If the tube is damaged then the bag will fill rather than empty.✻

The occlusion test✻
Occlude the lumen of the inner tube at the patient end✻ and look for dipping of the flowmeter bobbins✻✻ due to back pressure.✻

# Question 4

What are the special considerations required when anaesthetising a patient with carcinoid syndrome for removal of a gastric tumour? (90%)

## Answer
Carcinoid tumours are neuroendocrine✻ neoplasias usually originating from entero-chromaffin cells.
They are more common than previously thought (8% of autopsies). Ninety per cent are found in the gastrointestinal tract✻ although they may be found in many other sites such as the bronchus or gonads.
They are usually indolent✻ and the patient is asymptomatic.✻
If symptoms do occur they commonly present with abdominal pain,✻ diarrhoea,✻ GI obstruction✻ and bleeding,✻ or from the mechanical effects of tumours.✻✻
They commonly secrete serotonin✻✻ but this is metabolised on first pass through the liver.✻
Treatment options for symptomatic patients are excision, chemotherapy, or biotherapy with octreotide and interferon.✻

Fifteen per cent of patients with carcinoid tumours suffer from carcinoid syndrome.✻ Neuropeptides and amines are secreted into the systemic circulation.✻ Usually due to lung or liver metastases.✻

The patient is symptomatic of neuropeptides because they are released either without going through the portal circulation✶ or at such a high level that they overwhelm the liver's capacity to metabolise them all.✶

Carcinoid tumours may secrete serotonin, histamine, bradykinin, tachykinin, motilin, substance P, kallikrein, prostaglandins, catecholamines and other bio-active compounds.✶✶

Common symptoms include hypo-✶✶ or hypertension,✶✶ flushing, bronchoconstriction,✶✶ diarrhoea and carcinoid heart disease.✶✶

In carcinoid heart disease, the patient develops thickened valves and chordae resulting in tricuspid and pulmonary regurgitation and pulmonary stenosis (and more rarely mitral and aortic insufficiency).✶ Also pericarditis or myocardial metastases may occur. Treatment for carcinoid syndrome may include surgical resection or debulking, but is also pharmacological.✶ Cardiopulmonary effects are managed acutely with octreotide intravenously,✶ and chronically with long-acting depot somatostatin analogues✶ such as lanreotide.

The patient may have chronic pain✶ from their tumour or marked weight loss.✶
Check LFTs and U+Es preoperatively.✶
Avoid drugs releasing histamine (thiopentone, suxamethonium, atracurium).✶
Avoid catecholamines.✶
Invasive cardiovascular monitoring is usually required (arterial line, central venous cannula + or – transoesophageal echo).✶
Monitor electrolytes and glucose interoperatively.✶
Regional anaesthesia is controversial due to hypotension.
The mainstay treatment is intravenous octreotide for both prophylaxis and interoperative crises such as bronchospasm or low blood pressure.✶✶
If tumour is gastric, give prophylactic antihistamines.✶
Vasoactive drugs may produce crises. A test dose is advisable.✶
Historically, ketanserin, methysergide, cyproheptadine and aprotonin were used.
Postoperatively, continue haemodynamic monitoring, ensure effective analgesia, continue octreotide✶ and give ondansetron✶ for PONV.

### Reference
Dierdorf SF. Carcinoid tumour and carcinoid syndrome. *Curr Opin Anaesthesiol* 2003; **16**: 343–7.

## Question 5
In patients with chronic liver disease undergoing anaesthesia:
a) What are the relevant physiological changes which must be considered? (60%)
b) What pharmacological considerations affect the choice of neuromuscular blocker? (30%)

### Additional Notes
This question covers a lot of what you are expected to know about liver disease whilst also tying in some basic science. Below is presented an answer longer than you would be expected to write in the exam. This level of detail is here to provide you with a reference resource; the stars will guide you to the most important points.

Subdividing your answer into hepatic and non-hepatic will show clarity of thought to the examiner.

### Answer
a) Liver failure is characterised by the triad of:
    Jaundice✶✶
    Encephalopathy✶✶
    Coagulopathy✶✶

Hepatic:

Metabolic failure

Carbohydrate metabolism and glycogen regulation fails, resulting in hypoglycaemia, exaggerated with starvation.★★

Amino acid metabolism is altered, resulting in accumulation of ammonia and encephalopathy.

Cerebral oedema may occur in the acute (or acute on chronic) phase.

A poor nutritional state is often seen.★★

Synthetic failure

Protein – resulting in coagulopathy, hypoalbuminaemia.★★

Detoxification failure

Bile – jaundice.★★

Hormone – cortisol, oestrogen, aldosterone, ADH and thyroxine producing many of the sequelae of liver failure.★

Drugs – failure of phase I metabolism leads to prolonged and exaggerated action.★★

Storage failure

Glycogen – hypoglycaemia.★★

Vitamin – A, D, K, B12 and folate producing anaemia, coagulopathy and central neurological sequelae.

Extrahepatic:

Cardiovascular

Cardiomyopathy.★★

High cardiac output secondary to portapulmonary and spider angiomatous shunts.★★

Low SVR.★★

Depression of myocardial conduction by bile salts may result in third degree heart block after induction of anaesthesia.

The cardiomyopathy may only become apparent with the increase in SVR seen on intubation or during surgery.★

Respiratory

Intrapulmonary shunting produces VQ mismatch.★★

Hypoxic pulmonary vasoconstriction is impaired.

Together this results in hypoxia.★★

Pleural effusions and ascites reduce the FRC.★★

Haematological

Anaemia.★★

Thrombocytopaenia, impaired platelet function and clotting factor deficiency all contribute to coagulopathy.★★

Renal

Secondary hyperaldosteronism results in sodium and water retention and apparent hyponatraemia,★ which if inappropriately corrected may lead to central pontine myelinolysis.

Diuretic therapy may produce further electrolyte imbalance and intravascular volume depletion.

Hepatorenal syndrome★★ carries a mortality of over 90% and is related to renal hypoperfusion in the presence of jaundice.

Central nervous system

Encephalopathy.★★

Raised ICP is more commonly associated with acute liver failure.

Gastrointestinal

Portal hypertension and varices risk bleeding. Their management with β-blockers limits the cardiovascular response.★

Gastric reflux is more common.★

b) Pharmacological considerations when selecting a neuromuscular blocker in chronic liver disease:

Depolarising

Reduced plasma pseudocholinesterase prolongs the action of suxamethonium and mivacurium. ★★

Non-depolarising

These are water-soluble drugs which are poorly protein-bound.

Their $V_d$ therefore increases ★★ but their unbound portion changes by only a small percentage with the hypoalbuminaemia seen in liver disease.

There is therefore an apparent resistance to non-depolarising agents.

This phenomenon is, however, offset by a reduction in hepatic metabolism of steroid-based drugs (e.g. vecuronium). ★★ The fall in P450 activity and therefore phase I metabolism can mean that their duration of action may be extremely prolonged. ★★ Phase II metabolism is, however, unaltered. ★

Forty per cent of a dose of atracurium and cisatracurium undergo Hoffman degradation, therefore the elimination of these drugs is less dependent on hepatic clearance, making them the non-depolarising agents of choice. ★★

## Reference

Clarke P, Bellamy MC. Anaesthesia for patients with liver disease. *Contin Educ Anaesth Crit Care Pain* 2000; **4**: 158–61.

## Question 6

a) Give a definition of delirium as applied to a patient on a critical care unit. (10%)
b) List the causes of delirium in a patient on a critical care unit. (40%)
c) How may the incidence of delirium be kept to a minimum in a critical care unit? (40%)

## Additional Notes

This is a bit of a monster of a question so it is important to be succinct in your answer. Delirium in the critically ill occurs in 15–80% of patients depending on definition and is an independent predictor of mortality and increased length of stay. Delirium can be mistaken for, or found in combination with, other forms of mental illness, e.g. dementia, depression and psychosis. There are well-validated delirium screening tools, e.g. CAM-ICU (confusion assessment method for the intensive care unit) and the ISDSC (intensive care delirium screening checklist).

## Answer

a) Defined as 'an acute, ★★ reversible, ★ organic, ★★ mental syndrome ★ with disorders of attention ★ and cognitive function, ★ increased or decreased psychomotor activity ★ and a disordered sleep-wake cycle ★'.

Delirium can be further subdivided into three main subtypes: hyperactive, hypoactive and mixed (a combination of the first two).

b) Due to the complexity of this patient group there may be multiple causes. ★

The presence of dementia increases the risk of delirium 2–3 times. ★

Increasing age and low IQ are also risk factors, possibly due to low cognitive reserve. ★

Accurate history-taking is essential in helping to narrow down a likely cause. ★

Cerebral causes

Head injury ★

Cerebrovascular events, ★★ e.g. CVA, ★ cerebral abscess, seizures ★ (may be sub-clinical, therefore difficult to detect).

Metabolic causes
Fluid★ and electrolyte★★ abnormalities, acid-base disturbances★ and hypoxia★★
Hypoglycaemia★★
Hepatic★ or renal★ failure
Vitamin deficiency states (especially thiamine and cyanocobalamin)
Endocrine abnormalities, e.g. hypothyroidism

Hypoperfusion causes
Shock★★ (all causes)
Heart failure
Cardiac arrhythmias
Anaemia

Infectious causes★★
Urinary tract infection,★★ pneumonia,★★ meningitis★

Drug causes
Medication-induced delirium★★
    Drug side effects (mainly excess antimuscarinic and dopaminergic activity)
    Drug interactions
    Corticosteroids
Substance withdrawal,★★ e.g. from alcohol, opioids or benzodiazepines
Substance intoxication
Drug interactions

Other causes
Unfamiliar environment★★
Pain★
Hypothermia★

c) Prevention of delirium is more effective than treatment.★ Maintenance of the orientation of the patient to their surroundings and maintenance of normal physiological function are key.★★
Environmental and patient factors:
Maintain day/night cycle where possible★
Keep excessive noise to a minimum★
Deliver care to allow maximum uninterrupted sleep if possible★
Constant reminders of day, time, location and identity and role of carers★
Familiar objects from the patient's home may help★
Consistency of nursing care (same nurses where possible and maintenance of similar routine)★
Involvement of patient's relatives★
Use of television and radio to maintain link with 'outside world'★
Ensure glasses and hearing aids are used★
Encourage self-care where appropriate★

Minimising precipitants
Regular review of drug charts to minimise drug use★
Prompt identification and treatment of hypoxia, acidosis, hypo/hyperthermia, haemodynamic instability.★★

## References

Detection, prevention and treatment of delirium in critically ill patients. UKPCA. Online at http://www.ics.ac.uk/icmprof/downloads/UKCPA%20Delirium%20Resource%20June%202006%20v1%202.pdf (Accessed on 30 December 2008.)

Cohen I, Gallagher J, Pohlman A, Dasta J, Abraham E, Papadokos P. Physiology, pathophysiology and differential diagnosis of ICU agitation. *Crit Care Med* 2002; **30**: S98–S101.

## Question 7

a) What are the clinical features of critical illness polyneuropathy (CIPN)? (30%)
b) List the predisposing factors. (20%)
c) How is it diagnosed? (20%)
d) What are the difficulties encountered when managing a ventilated, critically ill patient with this condition? (20%)

### Answer

a) CIPN is common (>50% adult patients on ICU more than 1 week, >70% of those with sepsis/multiple organ dysfunction syndrome).✶ The clinical features are:
Acute in onset✶
Symmetrical✶
Hypo/areflexia (lower motor neurone pattern)✶✶
Motor and sensory polyneuropathy (although predominantly motor)✶✶
Extent of weakness proportional to duration of illness✶
Muscle atrophy✶
Respiratory muscle weakness✶
Legs affected more than arms
Relative sparing of facial muscles✶
Variable sensory loss (although difficult to assess in ICU patients)
Almost exclusively adults (usually >50yr)
Difficult to diagnose with certainty in many patients
Self-limiting

b) Predisposing factors for CIPN are:
Being ventilated✶✶ (for > 5 days✶)
Sepsis/SIRS✶✶
Multiple organ dysfunction syndrome✶✶
Incidence proportional to duration and severity of illness✶
Males
>50yr
Poor glycaemic control✶
Burns/trauma/surgery
Low serum albumin
Non-depolarising muscle relaxants, steroids and gentamicin have all been suggested as putting patients at risk of CIPN, but no definite link has been proven.

c) Diagnosis of CIPN involves identifying the clinical features✶✶ and risk factors✶✶ outlined above and the following investigations:

Nerve conduction studies✶✶
   Decreased action potential amplitude in motor and sensory nerves✶
   Normal conduction velocity✶

EMG✶✶
   Spontaneous muscle activity
   Fibrillation potentials and positive sharp waves are evidence of denervation injury

Nerve biopsy✲ shows
  Axonal degeneration
  Normal myelin
  No inflammation

Muscle biopsy✲ shows
  Denervation injury

d) Difficulties encountered when managing a ventilated patient with CIPN include:
  Prolonged time on ventilator✲✲
    Tracheostomies and the inherent risks of insertion and maintenance✲
    High risk of ventilator-acquired pneumonia✲
  Prolonged hospital stay✲✲
    Higher risk if develops nosocomial infections✲
  Disuse atrophy produces delayed mobility✲✲
  Pressure sores✲
  Venous thromboembolism
  Psychological problems such as depression or lack of motivation✲
  Dealing with family concerns and anxieties

## Question 8

a) Draw a waveform one would expect to see when transducing a central venous catheter inserted into an ASA 1 patient with a structurally normal heart. Explain which parts of the cardiac cycle cause the various undulations on this waveform. On the same diagram draw an ECG tracing showing the temporal relationship between the two. (30%)
b) List the factors that increase and decrease the central venous pressure. (20%)
c) What information can be gained from digital examination of an arterial pulse? (40%)

### Additional Notes

Core knowledge this one. Again, make sure you can draw and label and above all that you understand the basic diagrams that come up again and again in the exam. You need to think about the relationship between electrical activity and pressure in the heart as one can get confused in the heat of battle!

The last part is back to medical school finals. Think broadly to score all the available marks.

**Answer**

a) See Figure 6.

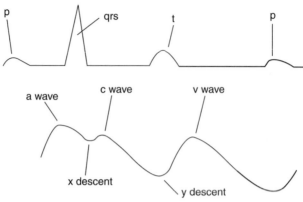

Central venous pressure waveform and ECG

Figure 6

The trace is made up of named waves and descents:

A wave from atrial contraction★★
C wave from isovolumetric contraction.★★ The 'notch' is due either to transmitted pulsation from the carotid arteries or to bulging of the tricuspid valve into the right atrium★
V wave from the rise in atrial pressure before tricuspid opening★
X descent represents downward movement of the right ventricle due to opening of the pulmonary valve, thus lowering central venous pressure★
Y descent is due to the tricuspid valve opening in diastole and blood emptying from the atria into the ventricle★
Showing p, qrs and t waves on ECG in correct position relative to pressure wave★

b) Central venous pressure is increased by either an increase in venous blood volume★★ or a decrease in venous compliance.★
    Raised intrathoracic pressure, e.g. IPPV or coughing★
    Venoconstriction★
    Impaired cardiac function, e.g. cardiac failure, tamponade★★
    Hypervolaemia★★
    Superior vena cava obstruction★

Central venous pressure is decreased by:
    Reduced venous return. Hypovolaemia can be relative, e.g. venodilatation,★ or absolute, e.g. haemorrhage or dehydration★★
    Reduced intrathoracic pressure (e.g. inspiration)★

c) A great deal can be gleaned from digital examination of a pulse.
    Rate★★
        Normal rate is 60–100bpm★

    Rhythm★★
        Regular (remember sinus arrhythmia is normal)★
        Irregularly irregular, e.g. atrial fibrillation★
        Regularly irregular, e.g. 2° heart block★

Volume*
Low, normal or high. Can be useful to compare volumes of different pulses, e.g. brachial and radial, as a measure of peripheral vasoconstriction as a surrogate for 'filling'. High-volume pulses seen in $CO_2$ retention, anaemia and thyrotoxicosis.

Character*
Best assessed at the carotid and refers to the pattern of the rise and fall of the pulse. Classic character pulses include collapsing (or waterhammer) seen in aortic incompetence or the 'slow rising' pulse of aortic stenosis.

Symmetry
Radioradial delay seen in aortic coarctation or radiofemoral delay also seen in aortic coarctation but more commonly seen in atherosclerotic disease.

Character of vessel wall
Atherosclerotic arteries may feel more rigid than normal ones.
Presence of bruits.
May be palpable as a thrill. Seen, again, in atherosclerotic disease.

## References

Ryder R, Mir M, Freeman E. *An aid to the MRCP Short Cases*. Blackwell Science Publications. 1986.
Gelman S. Venous function and central venous pressure: a physiologic story. *Anesthesiology* 2008; **108**: 735–48.

## Question 9

a) What are the cardiovascular effects of pregnancy at full term? (60%)
b) What physical manoeuvres can be performed to optimise cardiovascular function at the beginning of an elective caesarean section under regional anaesthesia? (30%)

## Additional Notes

There has been a paucity of obstetric questions in the Royal College Examinations over the past 8 years. This question incorporates maternal physiology with clinical practice and it therefore represents a reasonable FRCA question. The distribution of marks should guide you towards the expected content. Read the question carefully; there are no marks for an explanation of pharmacological agents in part b.

## Answer

a) Plasma volume increases by 45% but RBC mass by only 20%, leading to a fall in haemoglobin to 12g/dL (physiological anaemia of pregnancy).**
Total blood volume therefore increases by 45%.**
The vasodilatory effects of oestrogen and progesterone lead to a reduction in vascular resistance by 20%.**
SVR therefore falls from 1700 to 979dynes·sec·cm$^{-5}$.
This leads to a reduction in systolic BP by 6–8% and diastolic BP from 20–25%**
stimulating a baroreceptor-mediated reflex tachycardia with a rise in heart rate by 25% at term.*
The stroke volume rises by 25% facilitated by an increase in the ejection fraction by 20% and in the LVEDV by 10%.*
The combination of tachycardia and elevation in stroke volume results in a rise in the cardiac output by 50%.**

With the contraction of uterine muscle and the pain of labour, a further 15–50% rise in cardiac output may be seen.✶ This is associated with an increase in LV mass by 50%, but contractility remains unchanged.

The distribution of cardiac output changes such that the flow to the uterus, skin, kidneys, gut, breast and skin increases.✶✶

CVP, PAP and PCWP are all unchanged.✶

b) Consider this before siting the regional block.

Patient position

Establish regional with patient in full left or right lateral position (preferably left).✶✶

This minimises aortocaval compression and block height and therefore hypotension.✶✶

Only turn supine immediately prior to surgery and do so with left tilt of at least 15° – greater tilt may be beneficial; use the greatest amount of tilt the surgeon will tolerate.✶✶

Use table tilt, wedge or blankets.

The use of hyperbaric local anaesthetic solutions makes manipulation of block height possible through patient positioning. Thus a pillow limits cervical spread and therefore severe hypotension.✶

Fluid

The timing of fluid administration is important. Consider pre-loading and more importantly co-loading via a free-flowing 14 gauge venflon.✶✶

Rapid administration of fluid at the onset of sympathetic blockade may minimise cardiovascular instability.

## References

Power I, Kam P. Maternal physiology. In: *Principles of physiology for the anaesthetist*. London. Oxford University Press. 2001; 346–52.

Heideman BH, McClure JH. Changes in maternal physiology during pregnancy. *Contin Educ Anaesth Crit Care Pain* 2003; **3**: 65–8.

## Question 10

a) With the aid of the schematic diagram of a nephron show where the following classes of diuretic act, giving an example of each and briefly outline their mechanism of action.

Loop diuretic (10%)

Osmotic diuretic (10%)

Thiazide diuretic (10%)

Potassium sparing diuretic (10%)

Carbonic anhydrase inhibitor (10%)
See Figure 7

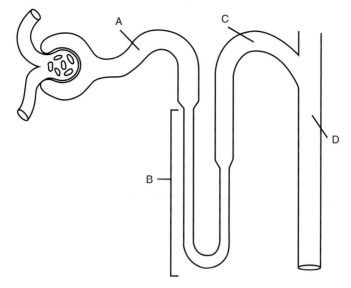

A Schematic Drawing of a Nephron

Figure 7

b) Discuss the potential risks associated with anaesthetising patients taking diuretics. (40%)

## Additional Notes

This is a classic question starting with basic pharmacology and then asking you to apply it to a clinical situation. With the new booklet format for the exam it would be easy for the College to insert diagrams that need annotating. The traditional way of asking this question would be to ask you to draw the basic diagram. Under those circumstances, remember that there are no marks for beautiful artwork – just marks for something that illustrates the point.

## Answer

A = proximal convoluted tubule (PCT). Site of action for carbonic anhydrase inhibitors.✶✶ Also loop diuretics have some action here.✶

B = loop of Henle. Divided up into descending limb, thin ascending limb and thick ascending limb. Site of action for the loop diuretics✶✶ such as furosemide which acts specifically on the thick (upper) part of the ascending loop.

C = distal convoluted tubule (DCT). Site of action of thiazide diuretics,✶✶ potassium sparing diuretics✶✶ and carbonic anhydrase inhibitors.✶✶

D = collecting duct. Site of action of osmotic✶✶ and potassium sparing diuretics.✶✶

Carbonic anhydrase inhibitors, e.g. acetazolamide✶✶

Work by reversible, non-competitive carbonic anhydrase inhibition.✶ This reduces the availability of hydrogen ions, which are usually exchanged for reabsorbed sodium ions in both the PCT and DCT thus promoting a diuresis.

Loop diuretics, e.g. furosemide✶✶

Work by inhibition of chloride ion reabsorption in the PCT and ascending limb of the loop of Henle.✶ By reducing interstitial hypertonicity and also by increasing renal blood flow without affecting glomerular filtration (and so reducing oncotic pressure) a powerful diuretic action occurs.

Thiazide diuretics, e.g. bendroflumethiazide✶✶
Act on the DCT by affecting the luminal membrane pumps so inhibiting sodium and chloride reabsorption.✶

Osmotic diuretics, e.g. mannitol✶✶
Pass freely through the glomerular basement membrane but are then non-reabsorbable once in the tubule. This increases the osmolality of the glomerular filtrate and tubular fluid so increasing urinary volume via an osmotic effect.✶

Potassium sparing diuretics, e.g. spironolactone or amiloride✶✶
Act as a competitive aldosterone antagonist✶ (spironolactone) or selective sodium reabsorption blocker✶ (amiloride) in the DCT. Net result is more sodium in the DCT and collecting ducts so promoting a diuresis.

b) When anaesthetising a patient on diuretics there are three main considerations:
Risk associated with the underlying medical condition.✶✶
Diuretics are prescribed for treatment of heart failure and hypertension so this should prompt further investigation preoperatively to look at these co-morbidities in more detail especially for evidence of end organ damage.✶

Risks associated with the diuretics themselves.✶✶
Diuretics have a number of side effects.
Electrolyte imbalances, e.g. hypokalaemia,✶✶ hyperkalaemia,✶✶ hyponatraemia,✶✶ hypocalcaemia and hypomagnesaemia.
Hyperchloraemic metabolic acidosis and metabolic alkalosis.✶
Interstitial nephritis leading to renal impairment (furosemide).
Bone marrow / haemopoietic problems.

Whether or not to omit diuretics in the perioperative period.✶✶
Due to fluid loss, reduced fluid intake and the vasodilating effects of most anaesthetic agents, diuretics are often stopped in the perioperative period.✶✶ Recommencement timing should be considered on a patient by patient basis.

## References

Brater C. Diuretic therapy. *NEJM* 1998; **339**: 387–95.
Sasada M, Smith S. *Drugs in anaesthesia and intensive care*, 3rd edition. Oxford University Press. 2003; 704–5.

## Question 11

a) List the ideal physicochemical properties of a volatile agent for use in the gaseous induction of anaesthesia. (30%)
b) Why is a gaseous induction in an 18-month-old child more rapid than one in an adult? (30%)
c) Why may upper airway obstruction slow this process? (30%)

## Additional Notes

This question tests your ability to combine basic science with the phenomena that you observe clinically… which is what anaesthetics is really all about. Many books claim that the high cardiac output of a child speeds gaseous induction. This is incorrect, but has been reprinted many times over. In fact, the opposite is true – don't fall victim to poorly written texts.

Try to construct a considered rational answer to part (c), supported with relevant formulae where possible; this illustrates a real understanding of the science and will score highly.

a) Physical:
   Pleasant to breathe.★★
   Non-irritant to the airways: no salivation, laryngospasm or bronchospasm which would slow induction.★★
   Cheap to produce.★
   Easily stored, long shelf life.★
   Non-corrosive to breathing system and anaesthetic machine.★★
   Safe with soda lime.★★
   Preservative-free.
   Not flammable or explosive.
   Environmentally friendly.

   Chemical:
   Low blood:gas partition coefficient.★★
   High oil:gas partition coefficient (low MAC).★★
   Potent enough to allow high $FiO_2$.★
   Easy to administer using standard vaporiser.★
   Vaporiser able to deliver high concentrations.
   Not epileptogenic, no cardiovascular compromise and no respiratory depression.★★
   Not metabolised, non-toxic, no allergic reactions.

b) Children:
   Have a higher alveolar minute ventilation ($V_A$) than adults (100 vs 60ml/kg per min).★★
   This results in more rapid approximation of inspired and alveolar agent concentrations, such that $F_A/F_I$ =5 minutes in a child, but 10 minutes in an adult.★★
   The ratio of alveolar ventilation to FRC in a child is much higher than in an adult – $V_A$/FRC=5:1 in a child, but 1.5:1 in an adult.★★
   These points result in a higher alveolar agent concentration in a shorter period.

   Once in the alveoli, the high concentration of agent has a more profound effect because children:
   Have a lower $V_d$ of lipid-soluble drugs.★
   Display an apparent reduction in blood:gas and tissue:blood solubility coefficients.
   Have a greater proportion of their cardiac output going to the brain.★
   Have an immature blood–brain barrier.★

c) Upper airway obstruction increases the turbulent airflow in the upper airways.★★
   The flow of gas (Q) in a turbulent system is given by:

   $$Q \, \alpha \, r^2 \frac{\sqrt{P_1 - P_0}}{\sqrt{l \cdot \rho}}$$

   where $r$ = radius, $P_1-P_0$ = pressure drop, $l$ = length and $\rho$ = gas density.
   The flow of gas (Q) past the obstruction therefore falls due to obstruction reducing the radius of the airway, the pressure drop not being linearly related to flow and increasing resistance to gas flow uncompensated by poor muscle power.★★

The reduction in gas flow has a detrimental impact on the first three values listed in (b) above:

1. $V_A$ falls, therefore less agent reaches the alveolus per minute.★★
2. $F_A/F_I$ increases, producing a longer alveolar equilibration time.★★
3. $V_A/FRC$ falls, diluting inspired anaesthetic agent with gas already present in the alveolus.★★

## Question 12

a) What is Parkinson's disease? (30%)
b) A 68-year-old male patient with Parkinson's disease is medicated with co-beneldopa (levodopa/benserazide) and cabergoline. He is scheduled for a laparoscopic cholecystectomy. What are the anaesthetic considerations specific to this patient? (60%)

### Additional Notes

Parkinson's disease is common in the elderly population. With this group of patients occupying an increasing proportion of your time, you should be familiar with the condition and the adjustments which you would need to make to your anaesthetic.

### Answer

a) Parkinson's disease is a disorder stemming from degeneration of the dopaminergic neurones in the substantia nigra and an imbalance of the dopaminergic/cholinergic central control mechanisms of the basal ganglia.★★
It is characterised by:
   Bradykinesia★★
   Tremor at rest★★
   Lead pipe rigidity★★
   Difficulty initiating movement★★
Other classic symptoms include monotonous speech, festinant gait, dribbling and micrographia.

b) The control of the patient's symptoms is dependent on the uninterrupted supply of anti-parkinsonian medication, which is only available in enteral form.★★ Significant decline in symptoms may occur with even one missed dose and the anaesthetist must try to address this.★★

Systemic considerations:
Respiratory
   Dysphagia, sialorrhoea and GORD risk pulmonary aspiration.★★
   Consider preoperative antisialogogue and rapid sequence induction.★
   Respiratory muscle incoordination, bradykinesia and sputum retention risk postoperative lower respiratory tract infection, particularly with atelectasis secondary to pneumoperitoneum.★★
   Consider postoperative respiratory physiotherapy ± high-dependency care.
   Mobilise as soon as possible postoperatively to reduce the risk of respiratory complications and DVT.

Cardiovascular
   Hypotension secondary to dysautonomia or drug side effects.★★ May be unmasked on induction and by pneumoperitoneum.
   Drug-induced arrhythmias can arise, especially with inhalational agents (not clinically significant).

Gastrointestinal

Reduced peristalsis will be exaggerated postoperatively.

Consider siting an NG tube to empty the stomach of gas prior to surgery and administer regular medication postoperatively (particularly if preoperative dysphagia which may worsen postoperatively).✱

Avoid antiemetics acting on the central dopaminergic system for fear of imbalancing parkinsonian control.✱✱ Use domperidone (doesn't cross blood–brain barrier), serotonin antagonists (ondansetron) or antihistamines (cyclizine).✱✱

Neurological

Postoperative confusion after GA is common; postoperative urinary retention is a potent catalyst.✱ Have a low threshold for catheterisation.

Avoid typical antipsychotics (phenothiazines/butyrophenones) should confusion develop – they worsen parkinsonian symptoms and may have extrapyramidal side effects.✱✱

Analgesia as per WHO analgesic ladder if no preoperative renal dysfunction. Involve the help of a neurologist specialising in Parkinson's disease, for advice on dose adjustment or medication alteration.

Laparoscopic cholecystectomy may not be a day case procedure in this patient. Admit and treat with care pre- and postoperatively.

## Reference

Teasdale A. Parkinson's disease. In: Allman KG, Wilson IH eds. *Oxford handbook of anaesthesia*. Oxford University Press. 2004; 176–9.

# Paper 3

Below are the model answers for this paper. ** indicates essential information, * indicates desirable information and unstarred text is supplementary information. As a guide, an answer with all the essential information and some desirable information would score 50% of the available points.

## Question 1

a) What are the anatomical relations of the tracheal carina? (50%)
b) List the indications for one-lung ventilation. (30%)
c) List the methods available for one-lung ventilation. (10%)

### Additional Notes

It is not mandatory to draw a diagram for an anatomy question unless it says draw. This question just asks for relations. The position of the carina is a complicated three-dimensional image that is difficult to draw well. Headed lists are perfectly acceptable for this answer.

The final part of this question is only worth 10% and should be very brief. The points available guide you as to what the answer should contain. This is simply a list of methods with no expansion into indications or techniques.

### Answer

a) The carina is the bifurcation of the trachea. *

It is at the level of the fourth thoracic vertebra or aortic arch. *
The last tracheal ring is larger and wider than other tracheal rings.
The orifice of the right main bronchus is wider and more vertical than the left.
The orifice of the left main bronchus is narrower and more angled.

The anatomical relations are as follows:
Anterior relations
  Mediastinal (tracheobronchial) lymph nodes
  Pulmonary arteries *
  Ascending aorta **
  Brachiocephalic veins/origin superior vena cava *
  Manubrium sternum *

Posterior relations
  Oesophagus **
  T4 vertebral body **
  Thoracic duct *

Left lateral relations
   Pleura and left lung∗
   Descending aorta∗∗
   Left recurrent laryngeal nerve

Right lateral relations
   Azygous vein
   Right recurrent laryngeal nerve
   Pleura and right lung∗

b) The indications for one-lung ventilation (OLV) can be divided into relative and absolute.∗∗

Absolute indications are:
Isolation of one lung from the other to avoid spillage or contamination∗∗
   Infection∗
   Massive hemorrhage∗
Control of the distribution of ventilation∗∗
   Bronchopleural fistula∗∗
   Bronchopleural cutaneous fistula∗
   Surgical opening of a major conducting airway∗
   Giant unilateral lung cyst or bulla∗
   Tracheobronchial tree disruption∗
   Life-threatening hypoxia due to unilateral lung disease∗
Unilateral bronchopulmonary lavage∗

Relative indications are:
Surgical exposure (high priority)
   Thoracic aortic aneurysm∗
   Pneumonectomy∗
   Upper lobectomy∗
   Mediastinal exposure∗
   Thoracoscopy∗
Surgical exposure (low priority)
   Middle and lower lobectomies and subsegmental resections
   Oesophageal surgery
   Thoracic spine procedure
   Minimally invasive cardiac surgery
Post-cardiopulmonary bypass after removal of totally occluding chronic unilateral pulmonary embolus∗
Severe hypoxia due to unilateral lung disease

c) Methods for OLV

Double-lumen endotracheal tube∗∗
Single-lumen endotracheal tube with a bronchial blocker∗∗
   Built-in∗
      Univent tube
   Isolated∗
      Arndt (wire-guided) endobronchial blocker set
      Balloon-tipped luminal catheters
Endobronchial intubation of a single-lumen endotracheal tube∗∗

## Question 2

After induction of anaesthesia in a 75kg adult for a routine case you discover that you cannot intubate or ventilate the patient. You have given 7mg of vecuronium at induction. A laryngeal mask airway (LMA) is not helpful. Describe what you would do next. (90%)

## Additional Notes

For this type of 'What would you do?' question, it is often helpful to think about what you would really do in your Trust. There is a vast array of different kit for trans-tracheal ventilation. A brief overview followed by a description of the one you are familiar with in your Trust is quite acceptable.

## Answer

This 'Can't Intubate, Can't Ventilate' (CICV) situation is an emergency and I would call for help.✭✭

I would remove the LMA and perform oropharyngeal suction,✭✭ then insert an oropharyngeal airway✭✭ and endeavour to perform four-handed bag and mask ventilation✭✭ with optimum head positioning and jaw thrust.✭✭ Some would maintain that the LMA should be left in situ as it provides a good airway for egress of gas following needle cricothyrotomy.

I would determine whether the problem might be laryngospasm by seeing whether it improved with further small IV anaesthesia increments.✭

If I still cannot ventilate the patient, I would now be looking to move to 'Plan D' of the Difficult Airway Society guidelines for CICV.✭✭ This involves rescue techniques to provide emergency oxygenation and should be instituted if the oxygen saturations have fallen below 90% on $FiO_2$ of 1.0.✭✭

The three styles of trans-tracheal airway are:

Small cannula techniques with a Sanders injector.✭✭
A patent airway is required for gas egress.✭✭ In one study, this was present in 86% of CICV patients.

Large cannula techniques (>4mm).✭✭
Lower-pressure ventilation but requires a cuffed tube or obstruction of the upper airway to achieve an adequate driving pressure. Many anaesthetists are adept at using these cuffed Seldinger-based kits (such as the Melker) as they are similar to percutaneous tracheostomy kits.✭

Surgical airway (6.0 to 7.0mm tube inserted).✭✭
This is easily taught,✭ has been shown to be quicker✭ in manikin studies, allows for sustained, adequate ventilation and has relatively fewer complications✭ than needle cricothyroidotomy.

Complications of these techniques may include malposition, false passage, haemorrhage,✭ oesophageal perforation,✭ surgical emphysema and barotrauma.✭

In our Trust, we have the Melker kit, which I would perform as follows:
The patient should have their neck supported in extension✭ and have their neck cleaned.✭
A cannula cricothyroidotomy✭ with the cannula provided in the kit is performed and confirmed by air aspiration.✭
The guidewire is inserted.✭
A horizontal skin incision is made.✭
The dilator is inserted over the wire and advanced.✭
The tube is inserted to the appropriate length.✭
A catheter mount and Ambu bag are attached and the patient is ventilated.✭
Capnography should be checked✭ and the chest observed and auscultated.✭✭
The neck should be examined for any signs of swelling during early ventilation.

If this fails, I would convert to surgical airway.✭

## Reference
DAS Guidelines online at http://www.das.uk.com/guidelines/guidelineshome.html (Accessed 1 January 2009.)

## Question 3

a) How does an intra-aortic balloon pump exert its physiological action and when might it be used? (45%)
b) What may be the reasons for a patient failing to wean from cardiopulmonary bypass following coronary artery bypass grafting? (45%)

### Additional Notes
Understanding the principles, complications and postoperative problems of bypass surgery and how to safely facilitate a patient's passage onto and off the circuit almost encompasses everything on which a fair cardiac question is based. Three such questions have been asked previously (1997, 1999 and 2002), but none has appeared since. Producing the diagrams shown below will show that you can incorporate first principles into your clinical practice – as ever label the diagram fully (✶✶).

The balloon pump question has not been asked before but still reflects core knowledge. Be prepared to draw an arterial pressure trace in a patient with an aortic balloon pump for both the SAQ and the vivas (not required here).

### Answer
a) Intra-aortic balloon pump (IABP)

This encompasses a double lumen catheter inserted via the femoral artery, connected to a console.✶

The inner lumen allows continuous blood pressure recording; the outer lumen allows for rapid inflation and deflation of a helium-filled balloon, which rests just distal to the left subclavian artery.✶

The balloon inflates as diastole begins, increasing diastolic pressure and therefore coronary artery perfusion pressure and in turn myocardial oxygen supply.✶✶

The balloon deflates as diastole ends, reducing left ventricular end diastolic pressure and afterload and in turn myocardial oxygen demand.✶✶

The IABP therefore increases $O_2$ supply and decreases $O_2$ demand.✶✶

Uses:

Acute MI (especially if associated with cardiogenic shock).✶✶

Unstable or impending acute coronary syndrome refractory to medical therapy.✶✶

During or post percutaneous coronary intervention.

Ischaemia-related malignant arrhythmias.

Refractory LV failure.✶✶

Pre or post cardiopulmonary bypass, or to assist weaning from it.✶✶

b) Reasons may be divided into:

Preoperative

Poor LV, ventricular akinesia, critical cardiac state.✶✶

Depressant drugs, e.g. calcium antagonists, β-blockers.✶

Perioperative

Heart

Preload

Inadequate, e.g. hypovolaemia, excessive blood siphoned into bypass circuit.✶✶

Contractility
Ischaemia, e.g. from inadequate cardioplegia (seen in ventricular hypertrophy), graft failure (graft kinks or air within the graft) or inadequate flow, e.g. insufficient perfusion pressure.★★
Native or prosthetic valve failure (stenosis or regurgitation).★★
Reperfusion injury.★
Afterload
Peripheral vascular resistance may be inadequate or excessive due to the use of vasoconstrictors and vasodilators.★
Pulmonary vascular resistance – see below.

Lung
Airways
Inadequate ventilation or $FiO_2$.★★
Barrier to gas transmission, e.g. bronchospasm.
Barrier to gas exchange, e.g. pulmonary oedema, atelectasis.★★
High pulmonary vascular resistance
Low $PaO_2$, high $PaCO_2$, acidosis, hypothermia, light plane of anaesthesia.★★
Inappropriate lung volume (see Figure 8).

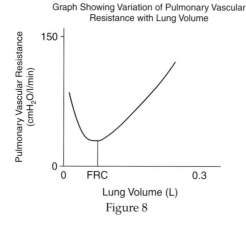

Graph Showing Variation of Pulmonary Vascular Resistance with Lung Volume

Figure 8

Low arterial or venous pressure (see Figure 9).

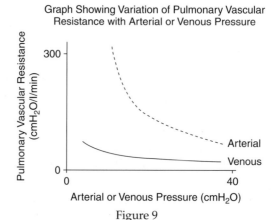

Graph Showing Variation of Pulmonary Vascular Resistance with Arterial or Venous Pressure

Figure 9

Hypoxic pulmonary vasoconstriction.✷
Drugs, e.g. vasoconstrictors.✷
Procedure
  Long bypass time.✷✷
  Long ischaemia time.✷✷
  Inadequate caridioplegia.✷✷
Blood values
  Electrolyte disturbance.✷
  Acid/base disturbance.✷✷
  Anaemia.✷
  Hypothermia.✷✷

## Reference

West JB. Blood flow and metabolism. In: *Respiratory physiology. The essentials*, 7th edition. Lippincott Williams & Wilkins. 2005; 35–47.

## Question 4

What measures would you employ to minimise the risk of central venous catheter (CVC) related infection in an intensive care unit you work in? (90%)

## Additional Notes

This is a big question and an example of thinking outside the box. It would be easy just to focus on the act of putting the line in but that would miss large chunks of mark-scoring opportunity. Remember a short question does not mean a short answer.

CVC-related infection is a hot topic. Approximately 3 in every 1000 patients admitted to hospital in the UK acquire a bloodstream infection and one-third of these are related to CVC use.

## Answer

Broadly speaking there are eight areas to consider:
Education✷✷
  There is good evidence that having a comprehensive staff-training programme on all aspects of CVC use reduces infection rates.✷ This should include regular audit of outcome data.✷

Aseptic technique✷✷
  This is essential when changing dressings✷✷ or accessing a CVC.✷✷ Hands must be washed using an appropriate antimicrobial solution.✷✷

CVC type✷✷
  Use a CVC with as few ports as possible.✷ Single lumen lines for long-term antibiotics or feeding are preferable to multilumen.
  Do not attach 3-way taps if possible as that just increases the number of routes for infection.✷
  If access is needed for more than 3–4 weeks then a tunnelled line is preferable.✷
  If insertion is in a patient at high risk of infection then a silver or chlorhexidine-coated or antimicrobial-impregnated catheter may confer benefit.✷

CVC insertion site✷
  When considering insertion site a balance needs to be struck between risk of infection and risk of mechanical complication.✷ In terms of infection

risk the subclavian route is probably preferable to the femoral or internal jugular.★

Insertion technique★★
It is essential to use maximal sterile barrier precautions when inserting a CVC.★★ These include gown,★★ mask,★★ sterile gloves,★★ cap★ and a large fenestrated drape.★

Skin Asepsis★★
Evidence suggests 2% chlorhexidine may be used to achieve cutaneous asepsis.★

Ongoing CVC care post-insertion★
The evidence for dressings is limited but on balance a sterile transparent dressing should be used to cover the CVC insertion site. There are a number of fixation devices recently on the market which may be preferable in the future. The skin should be cleaned with 2% chlorhexidine during dressing changes.★

CVC replacement strategies★★
Do not replace CVCs routinely to reduce infection.★
If a patient develops a CVC-related infection, remove the CVC and replace it at a different site.★
Keep CVC duration of use to an absolute minimum.★★

### Reference
Pratt R, Pellowe C, Wilson J, et al. Epic 2: National evidence-based guidelines for preventing healthcare associated infections in NHS Hospitals in England. *J Hosp Infect* 2007; **65S**: S1–S64. Available online at http://www.epic.tvu.ac.uk/PDF% 20Files/epic2/epic2-final.pdf

## Question 5

a) What pathological factors make a patient unsuitable for day case (12 hour stay)? (50%)
b) Discuss the use of regional anaesthesia in day case. (40%)

### Additional Notes
The examiner will have asked part (a) of the question in this way if they want to avoid you talking about the social factors that determine a patient's suitability for day case care. Do not mention social factors. You will be wasting your precious time and scoring no points. You may also lose marks for clarity. The surgical factors are relevant as they relate to pathology.

### Answer
a) Factors making a patient unsuitable for day case include:
General factors
Chronic disease that is poorly controlled/deteriorating or severe, i.e. ASA IV patients.★★
Class III obesity. Obesity is only a relative contraindication to day case surgery as patients with obesity who are otherwise fit and well having straightforward surgery may be suitable.★

Surgical factors
Body cavity surgery (i.e. laparotomy/thoracotomy)★
Potential major blood loss★

CVS factors
Poorly controlled/worsening ischaemic heart disease, including recent myocardial infarction.∗
Symptomatic cardiac failure∗
Symptomatic valvular heart disease∗
Symptomatic arrhythmias∗
Uncontrolled hypertension∗

Respiratory factors
Significant chest disease, including asthma, particularly if currently poorly controlled.∗

CNS factors
Recent TIA/CVA∗
Any severe disease, e.g. multiple sclerosis, myasthenia.∗

Metabolic
Poorly controlled diabetes mellitus (Type I patients with good control may be done as day cases).∗

Other systems
Significant renal/hepatic disease∗
Significant alcohol/drug abuse∗
Significant psychiatric disease∗

b) The use of regional anaesthesia in day case:
Peripheral nerve blocks are acceptable.∗
Patients can be discharged with residual block but the limb must be protected.∗
Central neural blocks are also acceptable.∗
Low-dose local/opioid mixtures are appropriate to minimise urinary retention and postural hypotension.∗
Use fine-gauge/pencil-point needles.
Requirements pre-ambulation are:
Not sedated∗
No postural hypotension∗
No hypovolaemia∗
Intact perianal sensation∗
Intact big toe proprioception∗
Appropriate leg motor function∗
The patient must void urine pre-discharge∗
Standard requirements also apply to patients receiving regional anaesthesia. Namely:
Well-controlled pain∗
Absence of PONV
Stable CVS/RS parameters∗
Responsible adult at home overnight
Must have private transport from hospital, available for use to come back if emergency
Phone at home
Written and verbal instructions to be supplied∗
Instructions to include information on duration of block∗
Oral analgesic drugs 'to take away'
Acceptable level of understanding∗

## Reference
AAGBI. Day case surgery. Feb 2005. 2nd edition. Currently unavailable online.

# Question 6

a) You are called to the emergency department to see a 40-year-old patient known to have taken an overdose of amitriptyline. What clinical features are consistent with an overdose of this nature? (40%)

b) In an adult patient with a history of paracetamol overdose, what investigations would you perform to determine the significance of the overdose (20%) and to monitor the patient's condition (30%).

## Additional Notes

Tricyclic antidepressant and paracetamol overdoses are common and may land patients on ICU. You would be expected to be familiar with their diagnosis and management. It is important to read the question carefully as in this case the management of these patients is not asked for. Such an answer will score no points.

## Answer

a) Features of tricyclic antidepressant overdose:
   From the history★★
      Previous overdose (OD)
      Depression with adverse life event
      Evidence of OD (empty packaging) or suicide note
      Patient volunteers information

   On examination:
   Cardiovascular
      Sinus tachycardia, dose-dependent long QT and widening of the QRS complex (the width of which is related to the severity of the overdose).★★
      Ventricular arrhythmias (especially if QRS >0.16secs or with acidosis).★★
      Right bundle branch block and right axis deviation.★
      Hypo- or hypertension.★★ Hypotension may be postural.
      Massive OD associated with hypotension progressing to PEA.★
   Neurological
      Excitation, seizures then falling conscious level and respiratory depression.★★
      Hyperreflexia and extensor plantars.★
      Divergent strabismus, convulsions.
      Abolished oculocephalic and oculovestibular reflexes.

   Anticholinergic
      Dry mouth, blurred vision and mydriasis, constipation, urinary retention.★★

b) Investigation of significance:
   Paracetamol levels 4 hours post-ingestion or immediately if unconscious.★★
   Levels >15 hours post-ingestion are unhelpful.
   Plot the level on the normogram, stratify the patient's risk as being normal or high risk and read off the appropriate treatment line.★★
   Significant OD if above the treatment line.★★
   Also check salicylate levels.
   Monitoring.
   Admit to acute ward or critical care as appropriate.
   Measure hourly urine output.★
   Do baseline liver function tests (bilirubin, AST, ALT, Alk Phos, albumin), glucose, clotting, arterial blood gas, urea, creatinine and electrolytes and measure daily, reducing to 12 hourly if significant OD (toxicity develops within 12 hours to 4 days post-ingestion).★★

The most sensitive marker and most useful prognosticator is elevation in the INR.★★ Elevation in ALT, AST and bilirubin suggests hepatic damage★★ (ALT is the preferred test on the NPIS 2007 guidelines – AST usually > ALT). AST and ALT >1000 IU/L represent paracetamol-induced hepatotoxicity.★ Significant decline and criteria for referral to a specialist centre include:

pH <7.3 (predicts mortality)★
INR >3 on day 2 or >4 thereafter★
Oliguria + increasing creatinine★
Decline in conscious level★
Hypoglycaemia★
Grade 3 or worse hepatic encephalopathy★

Factor V level less than 10% of normal = 91% mortality. Factor VIII to factor V ratio of less than 30 = 100% survival.

## References
Kumar P, Clark M. Drug therapy and poisoning. In: *Clinical medicine*, 5th edition. Saunders. 2002; 985–98.

## Question 7

a) The administration of multiple drugs in a short space of time means that anaesthetists are likely to make drug errors. How can this risk be reduced in the setting of a day case surgery unit? (40%)
b) How might the safety of epidural drug delivery for labour be improved? (50%)

## Additional Notes
Perioperative drug error has come under much scrutiny in recent years. This follows heightened awareness of the problem following improved critical incident reporting and information from national audits such as the Confidential Enquiry into Maternal and Child Health (CEMACH). The systems developed to reduce these problems are in varying stages of completion; some are still being conceptualised, others have now been incorporated into our daily practice.

You must be aware of the NPSA alerts relevant to anaesthesia. This explains the large number of essential (★★) statements in part (b).

## Answer
a) Incidence of drug error by anaesthetists: 0.75–4%.
  Preoperative
    Thorough preoperative assessment with note-keeping.★★
    Use of:
      Red allergy wrist bands are used by some trusts but are not recommended by NPSA.★
      Close communication with nursing staff regarding preoperative drug administration.
      Full patient check as in accordance with national guidelines.★★
    Review all of the above on the arrival of the patient in the anaesthetic room.★

  Perioperative
  The most important factor is anaesthetic vigilance.★★ Counterintuitively the presence of a second anaesthetist may require increased vigilance due to distraction or complacency.
  Draw up drugs for each patient individually.★★
  Careful checking of ampoules prior to drawing up drug.
  Do not administer a drug which has been drawn up by someone else.★

Use of standardised syringe labels and sizes (e.g. 5ml syringe for muscle relaxants).✲✲

Check each drug prior to administration with a colleague or using bar code technology.✲✲

Retain ampoules until patient safely recovered.✲

Ancillary drugs (antibiotics and local anaesthetics) kept away from general anaesthetic agents.

Organisational

Pharmacy to advise all anaesthetists if change in ampoule or packaging design. Increased use of:

Pre-loaded syringes.✲✲

Colour-coded infusion systems.

Dedicated connectors for all infusions.✲

'Smart pumps' which incorporate dose error reduction systems.

Ongoing use of critical incident reporting. A nationwide critical incident reporting system for anaesthesia is being developed.✲✲

b) Patient selection and infrastructure

Appropriate patient selection, investigations and consent.

Appropriate training of anaesthetists and midwives.✲✲

Close monitoring with standard physiological criteria, motor, sensory and pain scores.✲

Epidural equipment and drugs

Minimise likelihood of confusion between different solutions by:

Rationalising the range of injections and infusions available.✲✲

Maximising the use of ready-to-use infusions to reduce the risk of calculation or preparation error.✲✲

Storing epidural infusions separate from intravenous infusions.✲✲

Clearly label bags and syringes 'for epidural use only'.✲✲

Use of colour and design to differentiate these from other products.✲✲

Use lowest possible effective concentration of local anaesthetic.✲

Use clearly labelled infusion sets that are programmed for sole epidural use and are different from IV giving sets.✲✲

Used a closed system which should not be breached and an antibacterial filter.

Record-keeping, departmental guidelines and audit of the epidural service essential.✲✲

### References

Bowdle TA. Drug administration errors from the ASA closed claims project. *ASA Newsletter* 2003; **67**: 11–13.

Good practice in the management of continuous epidural analgesia in the hospital setting. November 2004. RCOA/AAGBI bulletin. Online at http://www.aagbi.org/publications/guidelines/docs/epidanalg04.pdf (Accessed 11 August 2008.)

Safer practice with epidural injections and infusions. NPSA patient safety alert. Issued 28 March 2007.

## Question 8

a) Briefly outline the uses of a fibreoptic bronchoscope in anaesthetic practice. (45%)

b) Once used for a percutaneous tracheostomy, describe the process by which the bronchoscope is made ready to be used again. (45%)

## Additional Notes

The fibreoptic bronchoscope has many uses both in theatres and on the critical care unit. If you use something then you should know how to clean it and as infection control is so high up the agenda at the moment it is a potential exam question.

## Answer

a) Uses can be broadly divided into diagnostic and therapeutic.

Diagnostic
Examination of trachea and major bronchi.★★
Examination of the oropharynx (nasendoscopy) as part of assessment of the potential difficult airway.★
As a diagnostic tool for biopsy or as part of a broncho-alveolar lavage (BAL).★★

Therapeutic
Removal of secretions.★★
Removal of foreign bodies.★
Re-expansion of collapsed lobes.★★
As part of endotracheal tube insertion either with the patient awake or asleep in the management of the difficult airway.★★
To check endotracheal tube position.★★
Particularly important as part of an endobronchial intubation, e.g. double lumen tube insertion.
To aid placement of a percutaneous tracheostomy.★★
Now considered part of a gold standard technique. Allows accurate cannulation of the trachea and also reduces complications.★

b) Cleaning a bronchoscope.
Always refer to the individual manufacturer's instructions★ and wear protective clothing when cleaning if splash contamination is likely.★
The cleaning process is divided into two stages, social cleaning★★ then disinfection.★★
Social cleaning (usually done by the anaesthetist):
Wipe down the exterior of the bronchoscope to remove any particulate matter.★
Remove and dismantle the suction valve for separate cleaning.
Clean the internal channel and port with a suitable cleaning brush.★
Flush the channel through with detergent or water.★
Following this and prior to disinfection all disposable parts should be removed and a leak test should be performed.★ If failed then the bronchoscope needs to be repaired before being used again.

Disinfection:
Can be carried out with glutaraldehyde, peracetic acid, chlorine dioxide, superoxidised water or ethylene oxide.★ Increasingly automated endoscope reprocessors are being used (AERs). These reduce the hazard of handling dangerous chemicals.
Whichever technique is used the bronchoscope must then be rinsed with sterile or bacteria-free water prior to use.★★
The bronchoscope must then be dried thoroughly★ and the process documented★★ before re-use.

## References

Mehta A, Prakash U, Garland R, et al. American College of Chest Physicians and American Association for Bronchoscopy Consensus Statement: prevention of flexible

bronchoscopy-associated infection. *Chest* 2005; **128;** 1742–55. Online at http://www.chestjournal.org/cgi/content/full/128/3/1742 (Accessed 28 December 2008.)
British Thoracic Society Guidelines on diagnostic flexible bronchoscopy. *Thorax* 2001; **56**:suppl I i1–i21.
Online at www.smartonweb.org/documenti/lineeGuida/Bronchoscopy.pdf (Accessed on 28 December 2008.)

## Question 9

An 18-year-old girl is ventilated on ITU two days following a road traffic accident during which she sustained a significant head injury (depressed skull fracture, bifrontal contusions and an extradural haematoma that has been evacuated). She has a cerebrospinal fluid (CSF) drain in and her intracranial pressure (ICP) has been stable but in the last hour it has risen from 10 to 30mmHg.
a)  Why might this have occurred? (40%)
b)  What sequence of management would you institute? (50%)

### Additional Notes

There are a lot of potential issues with this patient that you need to tease out to make a well-structured answer and there is a great deal of information to get across in your 15 minutes of furious writing. Lists or bullet points will help but 2 minutes of planning at the beginning to nail down a structure is recommended. Management of raised ICP is core knowledge but remember to read the question carefully as it is asking about specific management in her case rather than management of raised ICP per se.

### Answer

a)  There are a number of reasons why the ICP may have risen. These can be divided into primary causes★★ and exacerbating factors.★★ In this situation things to consider are:-
Primary causes
   Reaccumulation of extradural haematoma★★
   'Blossoming' of frontal contusions / cerebral oedema★★
   Cerebral infarction★★
   Developing hydrocephalus★★
      Blocked CSF drain★
      Incorrectly positioned CSF drain★
   Sagittal vein thrombosis (rare)
   New CSF infection (unlikely so early in history)
   Seizure (possible and may be difficult to diagnose in a sedated, ventilated patient)★★
   Measurement error, e.g. incorrect ICP monitor calibration★

Exacerbating factors
   Hypoxia★
   Fluid overload★
   Pyrexia★
   Hypercapnia★★
   Inadequate sedation/analgesia★★
   Uncoordinated ventilation★
   Inappropriate positioning★
   Iatrogenic obstruction to venous drainage, e.g. tight endotracheal tube tie★
   CSF drain set too high★
   Electrolyte abnormalities★

b) Management.

It is important to remember that it is a low cerebral perfusion pressure (CPP) and not necessarily a high ICP that will cause the damage so maintenance of CPP is of overriding concern✷✷ while the ICP is brought back under control by:

Identifying the underlying cause(s)

Treatment of underlying cause(s)

Removal of any exacerbating factors

Look at the patient to make sure she is well sedated and analgesed✷ (bolus doses of sedatives and analgesics may be needed), is not 'fighting' the ventilator✷ (a dose of muscle relaxant may be appropriate), is being nursed head up✷ and that the ICP reading is a true one.✷ Ensure an adequate blood pressure to maintain CPP. ✷✷ Examine the patient for evidence of seizure activity,✷✷ or infection✷ and make sure the pupils are equal and reactive.✷ Check temperature and cool if raised. Check that CSF is draining freely.✷ If not, DO NOT FLUSH DRAIN until appropriate imaging has been obtained.✷✷ Send a sample for MC+S if suspicion of infection. May be appropriate, depending on cause, to lower CSF drain height to allow more CSF to drain and so lower ICP.✷

Take a blood gas and correct any hypoxia and hypercapnia.

Alert radiology department about potential need for a CT scan and arrange transfer if diagnosis is unclear or patient does not respond to immediate treatment.✷ Remember that ICP control prior to transfer is ideal as patient needs to lie flat in scanner.

Other measures to consider in resistant cases are: boluses of hypertonic saline (NaCl 5%),✷ EEG to exclude seizure activity,✷ cooling (35°C or less),✷ thiopentone to cause burst suppression✷ (EEG monitoring essential) and decompressive craniectomy.✷

### References

Beed M, Sherman R, Majahan R. *Emergencies in critical care*. Oxford University Press. 2007; 182–91.

Girling K. Management of head injury in the intensive care unit. *Contin Educ Anaesth Crit Care Pain* 2004; **4**: 52–6.

## Question 10

a) How may humidity be defined? (20%)
b) List the devices used to measure humidity, describing the working principles of one of these in detail. (50%)
c) What is the clinical relevance of ensuring an appropriate level of humidity is obtained in the environment of a patient? (20%)

### Additional Notes

This is a compact topic, which lends itself to a SAQ. To avoid getting tied up in knots, use a mathematical description of humidity, as shown below.

The second part gives you scope to choose a device of your choice. Choosing the hair hygrometer would result in a very short answer and be unlikely to score as highly as a well-rounded description of another device.

### Answer

a) Humidity may be described in relative or absolute terms:

Absolute humidity =

Mass of water in a given volume of gas (units are mg/l)✷✷

Relative humdity =

$$\frac{\text{Mass of water in a given volume of gas}}{\text{Mass of water required to saturate the same volume of gas at the same temperature}}✷✷$$

(unit is %)

b) Devices
   Hair hygrometer✷✷
   Wet and dry bulb hygrometer✷✷
   Regnaults hygrometer✷✷
   Mass spectrometer✷✷
   Transducer✷✷
   UV light absorption

Wet and dry bulb hygrometer
   Two thermometers are used: one has a wet bulb wrapped in a wick, one has a dry bulb.
   Evaporation of water from the wet bulb results in cooling the thermometer (latent heat of vaporisation); the degree to which this occurs is inversely related to the ambient humidity.✷✷
   The disparity between the two temperatures recorded is read from tables to give a reading for the ambient humidity.✷✷
   A controlled air flow is required.✷

c) Relevance
   This can be subdivided into
1) Ambient humidity
   Too high is uncomfortable for staff; too low risks the adverse build-up of static electricity which may risk shock or, more likely, microshock to a patient.✷✷

2) Airway humidity
   Airway devices bypass the body's natural humidification mechanisms in the upper airway and anaesthetic gases are dry.✷✷
   This leads to artificially dry gas entering the trachea and bronchi directly.
   The adverse effects of this are:
      Humidification of the dry gas in the lower airways results in patient cooling (latent heat of vaporisation).✷✷
      Drying of the respiratory mucosa results in tenacious secretions. Impaired ciliary function compounds the problem, which risks mucous retention and infection.✷✷
      Surfactant function is also impaired, which risks atelectasis and pulmonary unit collapse, reducing FRC and increasing shunt fraction and hypoxia.✷
      Bronchoconstriction may also occur, causing difficulty in ventilation and worsening hypoxia.✷✷

### References
Davis PD, Kenny GNC. Humidification. In: *Basic physics and measurement in anaesthesia*, 5th edition. Butterworth Heinemann. 2005; 127–36.

## Question 11

a) What physiological changes occur when a patient is placed in the prone position? (30%)
b) What are the complications of anaesthesia in the prone position? (60%)

### Additional Notes
There have been recent reports of death or serious morbidity from patients being placed in the prone position and this subject has been well covered recently in a BJA editorial. You should therefore be familiar with the physiology involved and the risks.

## Answer

a) Physiological changes:

Cardiovascular

Rise in intrathoracic pressure which reduces both the venous return to the heart and the left ventricular compliance.★★

The resultant fall in the stroke volume reduces cardiac index by approximately 24%.★

Baroreceptor-mediated sympathetic output increases systemic and pulmonary vascular resistances and maintains mean arterial pressure.

Inferior vena caval obstruction raises venous pressure in Batsons plexus and may increase bleeding.★★

Respiratory

Functional residual capacity increases, coinciding with an increase in the $PaO_2$.★★

Traditional teaching is now challenged by evidence suggesting that perfusion remains dorsally distributed regardless of position.

More even distribution of ventilation results in improved V/Q matching and oxygenation.★★

Gastrointestinal

Increased intra-abdominal pressure and reduced venous drainage may impair perfusion to abdominal viscera.★★

b) Complications

Practicalities

Risks during turning:

Displacement or removal of intravenous or intra-arterial cannulae, central venous lines or the endotracheal tube.★★

Adverse events being undetected as monitoring leads are often disconnected at this time.★

Uncontrolled movement of the patient's limbs, neck or head resulting in injury.★

Injury to staff.

Whilst prone, usage and adjustment of all anaesthetic equipment and assessment of the patient can be more difficult.★

Injury by system

Central nervous

Arterial or venous occlusion, air entrainment or traction can produce cerebrovascular events, or spinal cord lesions.★

Peripheral nervous

Ocular – post operative visual loss from direct pressure raising intraocular pressure, reduced perfusion pressure, increased venous pressure or a combination.★★

Corneal abrasions.★★

Nerve – at risk include supraorbital, lingual, buccal, brachial plexus and its branches, lateral cutaneous nerve of the thigh and sciatic.★★

Airway

Reduced venous drainage produces macroglossia, oropharyngeal and salivary gland swelling.★

Together with tracheal compression, this may lead to airway obstruction on extubation.★★

Cardiovascular/perfusion

Direct arterial compression and increased venous pressure impairs oxygen delivery, increases venous bleeding and predisposes to compartment syndrome and rhabdomyolysis. The liver, pancreas and femoral head may be at particular risk of ischaemia via these mechanisms.★★

Mediastinal or right ventricular compression may further impair cardiac function beyond that described above.

Embolic phenomena, especially air.

### Reference

Edgcombe H, Carter K, Yarroe S. Anaesthesia in the prone position. *BJA* 2008; **100**: 165–83.

## Question 12

Classically, a new drug will undergo four phases of clinical trials in humans.
a) Briefly outline the purpose of each of these phases. (40%)
The Committee on Safety of Medicines produces a yellow card to be submitted in the event of an adverse drug reaction.
b) Under what circumstances would you fill in a yellow card? (50%)

### Answer

a) Phase I Trials: To assess safety,★★ tolerability,★ pharmacokinetics★ and pharmacodynamics★ at therapeutic doses★★ in humans.★★ May also involve incremental escalation to find the best dose.★

Phase II Trials: Once safety confirmed in Phase I trials, Phase II trials are used to determine how well a drug works.★★ There is sometimes some crossing over between Phase I and II in testing safety, efficacy and dosing.

Phase III Trials: These are usually large, multi-centred, randomised, controlled trials.★★ They should give the definitive answer as to how well a drug compares to the current therapeutic 'gold standard'.★

Phase IV Trials: This is the post-marketing surveillance phase.★★ This phase of pharmacovigilance is designed to pick up rare★ or delayed★ effects in a large population once the drug has been launched into routine clinical use★.

b) The yellow card scheme was introduced in 1964 to allow a doctor or dentist to report a suspicion that a drug may have harmed a patient.★★

A yellow card should be filled in if you suspect an adverse reaction is due to a drug★★ or combination of drugs,★ including blood products, radiographic contrast media, vaccines, herbal remedies and self-prescribed medicines.

Intensively monitored drugs are marked in the BNF with an inverted black triangle (▼).★★ In this group, all adverse drug reactions (ADRs) should be reported even if not considered serious.★★

For established drugs, all serious★★ ADRs in adults and all★★ ADRs in children (under 18 years) should be reported.

Other areas of particular concern for the yellow card scheme include when the reaction is delayed,★★ when the reaction is in the elderly population★★ or when the reaction may have caused congenital abnormalities.★★

You do not have to be certain about causality.★

If in any doubt, you should still submit a yellow form.★★

### Reference

http://yellowcard.mhra.gov.uk/ (Accessed 24 December 2008.)

# Paper 4

Below are the model answers for this paper. ✶ ✶ indicates essential information, ✶ indicates desirable information and unstarred text is supplementary information. As a guide, an answer with all the essential information and some desirable information would score 50% of the available points.

## Question 1

When a person donates a 'pint of blood' this is converted into a number of different blood products.

a) What are these products, what are they usually stored in and at what temperatures? (30%)
b) State what is contained in cryoprecipitate and list transfusion triggers for platelet transfusion. (20%)
c) How is a crossmatch carried out in the laboratory? (40%)

### Additional Notes

A blood donor can donate blood in one of two ways: either donating 'whole blood', which is then processed and separated later, or 'component donation', where the donor is attached to a cell separator that separates whole blood into its constituent parts, removes the required component and then returns the rest to the donor. As an anaesthetist you need to know how blood is stored, and transfusion triggers have been consistent frontline medical news for a few years now.

Even though this question is broken into (a), (b) and (c), it does, in fact, have six parts. Make sure you have answered them all.

### Answer

a) Whole blood is separated into
    Blood components
        Red cell concentrates ✶ ✶
        Platelet concentrates ✶ ✶
        Fresh plasma ✶ ✶
        Cryoprecipitate ✶ ✶
    Plasma derivatives
        Albumin ✶
        Coagulation factors ✶
        Immunoglobulin

At donation the donor blood is drawn into a plastic pack containing an anti-coagulant preservative solution, usually citrate phosphate dextrose✶✶ (CPD) or CPDA$_1$ (CPD + adenine✶). The citrate binds calcium and acts as an anticoagulant and the dextrose and adenine support red cell metabolism during storage.✶

Blood products are stored at the following temperatures:

| | |
|---|---|
| Cryoprecipitate | −20°C✶✶ |
| FFP | −20°C✶✶ |
| Albumin | Room temperature |
| Platelets | Room temperature✶ |
| Packed red cells | 4°C✶✶ |

b) Cryoprecipitate provides therapeutic amounts of factor VIII,✶ factor XIII,✶ von Willebrand factor, fibronectin and fibrinogen.✶✶

Reasonable clinical practice is to transfuse enough platelets to maintain the platelet count >10 × 10$^9$/L in stable non-bleeding patients,✶ >20 × 10$^9$ in unstable non-bleeding patients✶ and >50 × 10$^9$/L in bleeding patients or in those undergoing invasive procedures.✶

c) There are three main steps to a crossmatch and the technique relies on the fact that if red cells have serum added to them that contains antibody against them then agglutination of the red blood cells will occur.✶✶

Step 1. The recipient's blood is tested against serum of known identity to identify ABO group and Rhesus status.✶✶

Step 2. The recipient's blood is then screened for atypical antibodies against other groups, e.g. Kelly, Duff, Kidd.✶✶

Step 3. Recipient's serum is then matched to potential donor units, a sample from each being tested against this serum, so completing the full cross match. This testing is necessary to eliminate the risk of rare anti-bodies that were not screened for in step 2 reacting with the recipient's blood.✶

## References

Transfusion guidelines online at http://www.transfusionguidelines.org.uk (Accessed 1 January 2009.)
Strauss R. Pretransfusion trigger platelet counts and dose for prophylactic platelet transfusions. *Curr Opin Hematol* 2005; **12(6)**: 499–502.

## Question 2

a) List the factors leading to a delay in the start of a theatre list. (40%)
b) How might the efficiency of a theatre list be improved? (50%)

## Additional Notes

The temptation here may be to go for the Nobel laureate approach and vent one's spleen with an essay on the late theatre start. Do not be tempted. The list or bullet point approach takes less time to write and is easier to mark. It is worth noting that an inefficient theatre list may be a function of many factors and in some cases has little to do with the theatre environment itself.

**Answer**

a) The vast majority of delays in theatre can be circumvented by good leadership, a strong team ethic and above all excellent communication. This can break down for a number of reasons.

Delays can be categorised into:

Patient factors

Patient unfit for surgery ✶
Patient failing to attend on morning of surgery ✶
Operation not required ✶
Patient arriving late on morning of surgery ✶

Staffing factors

Surgeon unavailable ✶
Anaesthetist unavailable ✶
Scrub staff unavailable ✶
Lack of availability of porters ✶

Environmental factors

Outside the theatre suite
Unavailability of ward beds ✶
Unavailability of ITU/HDU facility postoperatively ✶
Failure to follow preoperative protocols, e.g. nil by mouth times ✶
Lack of adequate preoperative assessment facilities ✶
Lack of ward staff availability ✶
Inside the theatre suite
Overrunning of previous list ✶
Need for emergency case to interrupt list ✶
Equipment failure or unavailability ✶
Postoperative recovery unit full ✶

b) Ways to improve theatre list efficiency

It is important to note that an inefficient theatre list may be a function of a hospital-wide problem ✶ rather than a local issue, as list efficiency is dependent on a huge range of surrounding resources. ✶ There also needs to be a realistic assessment of what can and cannot realistically be achieved on any given theatre list. ✶ However, ways to improve list efficiency within the theatre environment itself include:

Knowing what is on the list and having early access to patient notes may reduce day-of-surgery cancellations and improve efficiency. ✶
Allowing adequate time for the anaesthetist and surgeon to assess any same-day-of-admission cases so scheduled start time must be appropriate. ✶
Provision of holding bays so patients can be sent for, checked in and even have lines or nerve blocks placed prior to coming to theatre. ✶
Team briefings at the start of each list to check and plan ahead for any problems, e.g. equipment availability, specific patient issues. ✶
Having specific personnel regularly attached to a certain list may foster good team ethos and working conditions thereby promoting better efficiency. ✶
Instead of having a surgeon-based system have a case-based system whereby certain cases are attached to specific theatres to ensure more efficient use of capacity.
Have good communication systems in place with clear identification of who the leaders are and where they are based so the unexpected can be dealt with promptly.
Theatre usage should be documented and audited and that information examined to look for potential efficiency improvements. ✶ ✶

## Reference

AAGBI. Theatre efficiency. Safety, quality of care and optimal use of resources. 2003. Online at http://www.aagbi.org/publications/guidelines/docs/theatreefficiency03.pdf

## Question 3

a) What is digoxin and what are the indications for its use? (15%)
b) What is the mechanism of action of digoxin? (30%)
c) A 55-year-old patient is scheduled for an open right hemicolectomy. How might the preoperative discovery of atrial fibrillation on the ECG change your approach to this patient's anaesthetic? (45%)

### Additional Notes

Digoxin is a commonly used drug and popular with examiners. With such a large percentage of the marks available for part (b), a comprehensive answer will be expected. The clinical scenario is a common one in everyday practice, making this an entirely reasonable question. Be systematic in your approach.

### Answer

a) Digoxin is a cardiac glycoside derived from the leaves of the foxglove.✶
   Indications:
   Rate control in supraventricular tachyarrythmias, particularly atrial fibrillation with rapid ventricular response.✶✶
   Inotropy in refractory severe heart failure.✶✶

b) Digoxin's mechanism of action is two-fold:
   Direct action.
   Competes with potassium for the binding site of the Na/K ATPase in myocardial cells.✶✶
   Inhibition of this pump results in increased intracellular concentrations of sodium, which are then exchanged for calcium at the Na/Ca counter-transporter.✶✶
   The net result of this process is increased intracellular concentration of calcium, which increases inotropy, excitability and the refractory periods of the AV node and bundle of His.✶

   Indirect action.
   Enhancing the release of ACh at the cardiac $m_2$ACh muscarinic receptors results in a vagal effect.✶✶
   This slows impulse conduction and prolongs the refractory period in the AV node and bundle of His.✶

c) The discovery of preoperative AF raises several questions which must be answered prior to anaesthetising the patient.

   Why is this patient in AF?
   Look to exclude:
   CVS – ischaemic heart disease, previous infarction, hypertension, heart failure, valvular disease (particularly mitral), endocarditis, cardiomyopathy.✶✶
   Resp – pneumonia, pulmonary embolus, bronchial carcinoma, sarcoidosis.✶✶
   Other – thyroid dysfunction, alcohol or illicit drug abuse, electrolyte imbalance, haemochromatosis.✶✶

Is the AF a marker for more significant cardiac disease?
   Check for diabetes

Does the answer to the first two questions result in impairment in the patient's exercise tolerance and ability to match oxygen demand with oxygen supply when the demands on his cardiovascular system are raised?

What is his anticoagulation status and what should it be?★★
   Is there atrial thrombus?

Does his overall risk of emboli warrant lifelong anticoagulation?

Plan:
   Directed history and examination★★
   Check FBC, clotting, U&E, Mg, Ca, TSH and T4, fasting glucose, LFT★★
   Urine dip
   CXR★★
   Refer to cardiologists for consideration of echo (with particular interest in LA size, presence of thrombi, function of mitral valve, regional wall motion abnormalities), exercise tolerance test and advice on anticoagulation requirements.★★
   Consider CPEX testing.

### References
Peck TE, Hill SA, Williams M. Anti-arrhythmics. In: *Pharmacology for anaesthesia and intensive care*, 2nd edition. London. Greenwich Medical Media Ltd. 2002; 221–39.

## Question 4

Concerning Do Not Attempt to Resuscitate orders (DNAR orders):

a)  Discuss reasons why a DNAR order may be implemented. (40%)

   An intellectually high-performing (IQ 135) 14-year-old with severe spasticity from cerebral palsy attending for contracture release has stated that should she have a cardiac arrest under anaesthesia she wishes not to be resuscitated. Her parents are adamant she should be.

b)  What are the specific issues that you would wish to clarify in your preoperative discussions and who else would you involve with specific reference to this issue? (50%)

### Additional Notes
This question is quite different from the majority you will face in the SAQ part of the final FRCA. This is in part because this sort of question is difficult to mark. However, the recent publication of the revised mental capacity act does make an 'ethical type' question more likely.

### Answer
a)  In essence, when making a decision whether or not to implement a DNAR order one is balancing the patient's right to life★★ with the rights of patient choice★★ and the right to be free from degrading treatment.★★ To write a DNAR order, the following issues should be considered:
   1.  That cardiopulmonary resuscitation (CPR) would be futile, i.e. very unlikely to succeed, or that if it did, the patient would not survive to hospital discharge.★

2. That even if CPR were successful the quality of life that would follow would not be in the best interests of the patient.✶

3. What the patient wishes after a full and frank discussion or based on the instruction of any advanced directives / living wills.✶ An accurately recorded and consistently expressed opinion from a patient will suffice – there is no need in law to have an advanced directive written down, though clearly this is the ideal.✶ Some patients may make it clear that despite the clinical judgement of the medical team they still wish CPR to occur. In these situations clinicians cannot be required to carry out any treatment against their clinical judgement but they should respect the wishes of the patient even if there is a very small chance of success or benefit.

b) Respecting the wishes of children.
This has the potential to be an extremely challenging and difficult interview.✶ Surgery should be postponed until the matter is fully resolved.✶✶
It would be vital prior to the interview to involve senior colleagues✶✶ including a designated doctor for child protection✶✶ and, if it is thought necessary, to seek the advice of the hospital's legal team✶ and ethics committee.✶ You could also speak with your own defence organisation. The main issues that must be clarified are:
What is in the child's best interests?✶✶
Does the child have capacity?✶✶

There may need to be a series of discussions both with the child on her own and with her parents, if that is possible.✶ The confidentiality of the child should be respected wherever possible, as should her reasons for her decision.✶
It is essential to assess the child's capacity to refuse treatment in this situation. Capacity is defined as the ability of a child to understand, retain, use and weigh this information and communicate this decision to others.✶ Before the age of 16 a child may well have the capacity to consent to and refuse treatment and parents cannot override the competent consent of a young person to treatment that you as a health professional consider is in their best interests.✶ However, the legal position in England and Wales means that, in some circumstances where a child has made a competent refusal of a treatment, a person with parental responsibility or the courts may nevertheless authorise treatment where it is in the child's best interests.✶

### References
0–18 years: guidance for all doctors. General Medical Council Publication. Pages 14–15. Online at http://www.gmc-uk.org/guidance/ethical_guidance/children_guidance/index.asp (Accessed 3 January 2009.)
Withholding and withdrawing life-prolonging treatments: good practice in decision-making. General Medical Council Publication. Points 67–77. Online http://www.gmc-uk.org/guidance/current/library/witholding_lifeprolonging_guidance.asp#Children (Accessed 3 January 2009.)

## Question 5

Describe the mechanism of action of the agents which may be used to artificially elevate gastric pH. (90%)

### Additional Notes
The ability to increase gastric pH pharmacologically is something which anaesthetists use on a daily basis. You should therefore be able to describe freely the drugs used commonly and their mechanisms of action. An extensive list of drugs alone

will score less highly than a shorter list with a thorough explanation of the intracellular mechanism of drug action as the question asks you to 'Describe...'.

As ever, try to be systematic in your approach and try not to forget the most basic drugs.

## Answer

1. Drugs acting within the stomach lumen
   Act by a physicochemical effect on stomach acid.
   As the stomach empties, their effect wanes, so have a rapid onset but short duration of action.
   Only administered enterally.

a) Aluminium- or magnesium-containing drugs★★
   Poorly absorbed; minimal effect on plasma pH, significant effects on gut transit times.
   Sucralfate protects the mucosa from acid-pepsin erosion in ulcer disease.

b) Sodium bicarbonate/citrate★★
   Rapid onset of action and easily absorbed; risks metabolic alkalosis.
   Chemical action may produce $CO_2$.

c) Alginate-containing drugs (e.g. Gaviscon)
   Rafting agents reducing reflux and protecting the oesophageal mucosa. Their effect on gastric pH is limited.

2. Drugs acting on the production of stomach acid
   Parietal cells in the body and fundus of the stomach are responsible for the production of hydrochloric acid.
   See Figure 10. '+' indicates stimulation, '−' indicates inhibition.

a) $H_2$ receptor antagonists★★
   E.g. ranitidine, cimetidine (less used due to inhibition of P450).

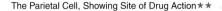

The Parietal Cell, Showing Site of Drug Action★★

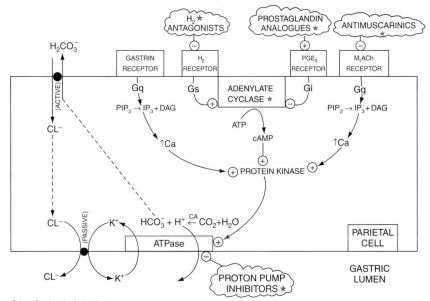

CA = Carbonic Anhydrase

Figure 10

b) Prostaglandin analogues★★

E.g. misoprostol (a synthetic analogue of $PGE_1$).

$H_2$ receptor antagonists act by blocking the stimulatory effect of $G_s$ protein; prostaglandin analogues act by propagating the inhibitory effect of $G_i$ protein, both of which reduce the activity of adenylate cyclase.★★

This reduces intracellular cAMP and therefore, via protein kinase, the action of $K^+/H^+$ ATPase countertransporter responsible for addition of $H^+$ ions to the gastric lumen.★

c) Antimuscarinics★★

E.g. pirenzipine

Antagonises the effect of ACh and the subsequent action of $G_q$ on $PIP_2$.★

The reduction in intracellular calcium slows the action of protein kinase on the ATPase countertransporter and therefore the amount of $H^+$ ions extruded.

d) Proton pump inhibitors★★

E.g. omperazole, pantoprazole.

Non-competitively block the $K^+/H^+$ ATPase countertransporter and therefore the final common pathway in acid production.★★

This results in complete achlorhydria and synthesis of new ATPase enzyme is required for acid production to recommence.

## References

Pinnock C, Lin T, Smith T. Gastrointestinal physiology. In: *Fundamentals of anaesthesia*, 2nd edition. London. Greenwich Medical Media Ltd. 2003; 455–71.

Power I, Kam P. Gastrointestinal physiology. In: *Principles of physiology for the anaesthetist*. London. Oxford University Press. 2001; 167–81.

## Question 6

a) How is lactate produced in the human body? (40%)
b) What are the causes of a lactic acidosis? (50%)

## Additional Notes

We frequently use measurement of lactate to guide our decision-making. You should therefore be able to explain what it is and where it comes from, even though this requires the use of some hard-core basic science.

## Answer

a) Lactic acid is a glycolytic by-product★ which can be produced by any tissue.★

Indeed, approximately 1400 mmol of lactic acid is produced daily. The vast majority of this is cleared either hepatically or renally.★

It is formed as follows:

The process of glycolysis converts glucose to pyruvate.★ Pyruvate is converted to acetyl-CoA (by pyruvate dehydrogenase), which enters the tricarboxylic acid (TCA) cycle.★

Glycolysis does not require oxygen, the TCA cycle does.★★

In hypoxic conditions the end products of glycolysis (pyruvate, NADH and $H^+$) accumulate, as pyruvate cannot enter the TCA cycle.★

To allow glycolysis to continue and therefore to maintain some ATP production, these end products are combined to form lactic acid; the reaction being catalysed by lactate dehydrogenase.★★

The lactic acid diffuses out of the cell into the extracellular fluid.★

By removing the end products of glycolysis in this way, the reaction can continue and useful (albeit reduced) levels of ATP can continue to be generated.★
When oxygen is re-supplied the lactic acid can be reconverted to glucose or used for ATP production by re-conversion into pyruvate, NADH and $H^+$.★
All tissues apart from red blood cells can use lactic acid for energy production in this way; the heart is particularly adept.★

Simplified view of glycolysis (anaerobic)
Glucose$\rightarrow$2ATP + 2Pyruvate + 2NADH + 2$H^+$★

The utility of these end products depends on the supply of oxygen.
In aerobic conditions:
$\rightarrow$2Acetyl CoA$\rightarrow$Tricarboxylic acid cycle★

In anaerobic conditions:
$\rightarrow$2 Lactic acid★

b) Blood lactate levels will rise if the rate of production overwhelms the hepato-renal capability to clear it from the body.★
Normal blood lactate concentration in unstressed patients is 0.5–1.0 mmol/L.★
Normal levels in critical illness <2 mmol/L.★
Hyperlactatemia is defined as a mild-to-moderate (2–5 mmol/L) persistent increase in blood lactate concentration without metabolic acidosis.★
Lactic acidosis is characterised by persistently increased blood lactate levels (>5 mmol/L) in association with metabolic acidosis.★★
Lactic acidosis can be congenital or acquired, the former being much rarer and generally secondary to inborn errors of metabolism.★
Lactic acidosis can be divided into two main types, A and B.

In Type A the lactic acidosis is due to an oxygen deficit which can be caused anywhere in the oxygen delivery chain and results in tissue hypoxia.★★ Causes of hypoxia may be hypoxic, stagnant, anaemic or histotoxic.★
   Causes of Type A lactic acidosis:
      Severe hypoxia★★
      Severe anaemia★
      Cardiac failure★
      Shock (all causes)★
      Severe exercise★
      Status epilepticus

In Type B lactic acidosis the problem is with lactic acid metabolism and not tissue hypoxia.★ Decreased lactic acid removal is usually hepatic in origin.★
   Causes of Type B lactic acidosis:
      Diabetes mellitus★
      Liver failure★
      Renal failure★
      Drugs, e.g. ethanol, ethylene glycol, salicylates, cocaine, theophyllines★
      Congenital causes, e.g. glycogen-storage disorders

## References

Luft F. Lactic acidosis update for critical care clinicians. *J Am Soc Nephrol* 2001; **12**: S15–S19. Online at http://jasn.asnjournals.org/cgi/reprint/12/suppl_1/S15 (Accessed 30 December 2008.)
Handy J. Lactate – the bad boy of metabolism, or simply misunderstood? *Curr Anaesth Crit Care* 2006; **17(1–2)**: 71–6. Online at http://download.journals.elsevierhealth.com/pdfs/journals/0953-7112/PIIS0953711206000585.pdf (Accessed 1 January 2009.)

## Question 7

a) Draw the view obtained during direct laryngoscopy of a Cormack and Lehane Grade 1 intubation. (40%)
b) List the possible causes and differential diagnosis of laryngospasm. (20%)
c) At the end of a case following removal of the endotracheal tube a 4-year-old child appears to go into laryngospasm. Outline your management strategy. (30%)

### Additional Notes

This should be easy but given the number of times you intubate someone in the years leading up to Final FRCA it is surprising how often a candidate struggles with a simple diagram. Practise drawing them – I went through the 'A to Z' (*Anaesthesia A to Z*, Yentis, Hirsch, Smith) before the exam and made sure I could draw and explain the diagrams in it. People with Da Vinci-level art skills do not get better marks so keep the diagrams simple.

The third part needs a structured approach. Remember to call for help. It will get a mark and is not a sign of failure!

### Answer

a) See Figure 11

The view obtained during direct laryngoscopy of a Cormack and Lehane Grade 1 intubation

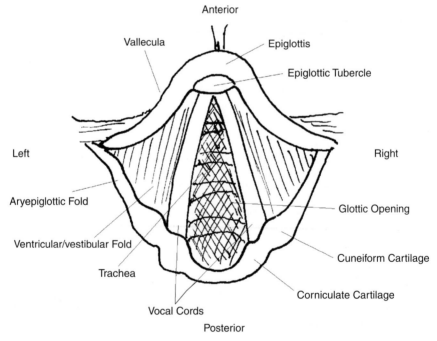

Figure 11

Will include:
A clear title
Orientation marks, correctly placed. Anterior, Posterior, Right and Left
Epiglottic tubercle★
Vallecula★★

Aryepiglottic fold✱
Corniculate cartilage
Glottic opening✱✱
Cuneiform cartilage
Vocal cords✱✱
Vestibular fold✱

Cormack and Lehane Classification
Grade I:    Complete glottis visible✱✱
Grade II:   Anterior glottis not seen
Grade III:  Epiglottis seen, but not glottis
Grade IV:   Epiglottis not seen

b) Causes of laryngospasm
Airway manipulation✱✱
Blood / other secretions in the pharynx✱✱
Regurgitation or vomiting✱✱
Surgical stimulus / inadequate anaesthesia✱✱
Moving patient✱
Irritant volatile anaesthetic agent✱✱
Idiopathic

Differential diagnosis
Bronchospasm✱✱
Laryngeal trauma / airway oedema✱
Inhaled foreign body✱
Tracheomalacia
Croup
Epiglottitis
Recurrent laryngeal nerve damage

c) Initial management
Aim is to maintain adequate oxygenation until the laryngospasm resolves.✱✱
Call for help early.✱
Switch to 100% oxygen✱✱ delivered with CPAP✱✱ if possible.
Eliminate precipitating cause✱✱ e.g. clear secretions, deepen anaesthesia, tell surgeon to stop.
Airway manipulation may be good or bad depending on the cause!
Beware hypoxic bradycardia so have atropine to hand.✱
Suxamethonium 0.25–0.5 mg/kg will relieve laryngospasm.✱✱
Reintubation and ventilation may be necessary.✱✱

Subsequent management
Watch for evidence of pulmonary oedema (so-called 'negative pressure' pulmonary oedema).✱
Remember to decompress the stomach, particularly after prolonged CPAP.
There is the potential for awareness in this situation so visit the patient on the ward postoperatively.

## References

Visvanathan T, Kluger M, Webb R, Westhorpe R. Crisis management during anaesthesia: laryngospasm. *Qual Saf Health Care* 2005; **14**: e3. Online at http://www.qshc.com/cgi/content/full/14/3/e3 (Accessed 30 December 2008.)
Allman K, Wilson I. Severe laryngospasm. *Oxford handbook of anaesthesia*. Oxford University Press. 2006; 842–3.

# Question 8

a) What are the physical differences between a re-usable laryngeal mask and an intubating laryngeal mask (iLMA)? (20%)
b) What are the indications for using an iLMA? (20%)
c) What would you do if your first attempt to intubate down an iLMA were unsuccessful? (50%)

## Answer

a) In comparison with a re-usable laryngeal mask airway (LMA), an intubating laryngeal mask airway (iLMA) has:
An epiglottic lifting bar.✷✷
No grille bars at the opening of the cuffed end.✷
A reinforced tube section✷ with a fixed curve.✷
An ergonomically shaped handle to aid insertion.✷

b) An iLMA should be used as the Plan B in a 'Can't Intubate, Can Ventilate' scenario once all your routine, simple intubation tactics have failed.✷✷
An iLMA may be used for planned difficult intubations where mouth opening is adequate but laryngoscopy is difficult.✷

c) If initial passage of the endotracheal tube through the iLMA proves unsuccessful, the first stage is to check that the iLMA is the correct size and well positioned.✷✷
A leak may indicate too small an iLMA.✷
A sub-optimal airway or the tube appearing high in the mouth or pointing in a caudal direction may indicate too large a tube.✷
The iLMA should have been initially deflated correctly ('boat' shape) and the patient placed in a head neutral position.
If any of these factors were of concern, they should be adjusted until satisfied with the position and ease of ventilation through the iLMA.
If the iLMA appears well positioned, the next tactic would be to have a second attempt at passing the tube.✷
If this fails, the iLMA should be deflated, withdrawn 6 cm into the upper pharynx, and then re-inserted. This may improve orientation between the epiglottis and the lifting bar.✷
If after attempting re-insertion you still fail to intubate, moving the iLMA in the sagittal plane to achieve optimal ventilation may aid successful passing of the tube.✷
If none of these blind techniques works, intubation may be aided using a fibreoptic scope through the endotracheal tube if available.✷✷ This may be used during initial attempts if available and likely to aid success.✷
Persistence with iLMA-based techniques hinges on safely ventilating the patient through the iLMA in between attempts at intubation.✷
In general, it is wise to limit the number of attempts at intubation to 2 before abandoning intubation via the iLMA, moving on to Plan C.✷✷

## References

DAS Guidelines online at http://www.das.uk.com/guidelines/guidelineshome.html (Accessed 1 January 2009.)

# Question 9

a) What criteria must be met for a patient to be considered for a Non-Heart-Beating Organ Donation (NHBD)? (25%)
b) Describe a timeline for an intensive care patient being considered for NHBD through to organ retrieval. (40%)
c) What advantages does beating-heart donation have over NHBD? (25%)

**Answer**

a) In the UK, there is published guidance:

    Age <70 years

    Multidisciplinary team decision on futility of treatment✷✷

    Assent from next of kin✷✷

    No HIV/AIDS✷

    No CJD

    Not active IVDU✷

    No recent malignancy✷

Final decision on inclusion between consultant transplant surgeon and consultant renal physician based on patient's past medical history and present condition.

b) The process:

    Is it appropriate to withdraw life support on grounds of clinical futility?✷✷

    Is the patient suitable for NHBD as outlined above?✷

    Is the patient on the Organ Donor Register? This is not mandatory, but is useful information going into discussion with the family.

    Approach the family.✷✷

    Activate the retrieval team.✷

    Withdraw support.✷✷

    If death takes >3hrs, stand team down (this time is variable from region to region but should be fixed pre-withdrawal).✷

    Cardiorespiratory arrest.✷✷

    Death certified at 5min.✷

    Time allowed for family goodbyes.

    To operating theatre for organ retrieval (usually kidneys and liver). A variation on this would be going to theatre pre-withdrawal.✷

    In the USA, insertion of femoral cannulae, pre-withdrawal inotropes and heparinisation have been performed.

c) Organ advantages.

    The downfall in NHBD is warm ischaemia time, which is very short in BHD.✷✷

    Lower incidence of delayed graft function✷ although long-term outcome is similar.

    Ethical and logistical advantages.

    Brain stem testing is a highly sensitive test of clinical futility with a definitive moment at which death occurs.✷✷ Apart from brain stem death, there is no legal definition of clinical futility as each patient is different.

    It is more widely accepted through many cultures which may have reservations about NHBD.

    In NHBD, the decision on clinical futility is less robust. Concerns remain about the 'Lazarus Phenomenon' in which a moribund patient rallies. Twenty cases reported since 1982.

    BHD does not have the conflict of interest inherent in NHBD.✷ The discussion about withdrawal and the discussion about organ procurement are separate.✷ In NHBD, they are intimately linked. This creates issues about whether all options have been explored or whether you are acting in the patient's best interests. In NHBD there is an imperative to keep the 'arrest-to-death' time as short as possible to enhance organ survival. Currently waiting for national guidelines on timing death.

**Reference**

Gardiner D, Riley B. Non-heart-beating organ donation – solution or a step too far? *Anaesthesia* 2007; **62**: 431–3.

Ridley S, Bonner S, Bray K, et al. UK guidance for non-heart-beating donation. *Br J Anaesth* 2005; **95**: 592–5.

# Question 10

a) What are the mechanisms bacteria use to gain resistance to antibiotics? (40%)

b) What clinical problems are typically caused by vancomycin-resistant enterococci (VRE) and what antibiotics would you use to treat a sick patient found to have VRE bacteraemia? (50%)

## Additional Notes

Oh dear. This is a real clanger of a question and one which will make some candidates want to leave the examination room. Lucky you bought this book and a model answer is provided below.

Hospital-acquired infections are very topical and you work on ICU, which is a hive for them, so some knowledge about them is advised. Actually the answer to this question is not that taxing, as you will see, so it is worth having it up your sleeve.

## Answer

a) Bacteria may be resistant:
    Naturally✶
    By single point genetic mutation✶
    By transfer of genetic material, which may be 'naked' DNA or via a bacteriophage (a viral vector) or plasmids✶✶

The mechanisms are:
Drug inactivation✶
    β-Lactamase.
Reduced drug permeability✶
    Loss of the OprD porin in *P. aeruginosa* to produce imipenem resistance.
Target modification✶
    Either by changing the target metabolic pathway (e.g. absence of cell wall), or reducing the susceptibility of the target protein (low-affinity penicillin-binding protein for methicillin resistance).
Drug efflux pumps✶
    The broad-spectrum cytoplasmic pump MexB in *P. aeruginosa*.

b) Clinical problems

1. The host
    VRE is common in patients who:
    Are immunocompromised✶✶
    Have been fed by NG tube
    Have been in-patients for long periods✶✶
    Have received certain antibiotics (particularly vancomycin, teicoplanin or cephalosporins)✶✶
    Therefore commonly seen in ICU, renal, oncology and transplant patients.✶

2. Clinical infection
    VRE behave like other enterococci and cause the same range of infections, typically urinary infections, bacteraemias or wound infections (where enterococci are the 2nd/3rd most-common pathogen).✶✶
    They are infrequently responsible for respiratory infections, cellulitis, osteomyelitis, endocarditis and meningitis.

3. Ease of transmission✶✶
    Soap hand-wash ineffective✶✶
    Viable on surfaces for weeks✶
    Resistant to desiccation and extreme temperatures✶✶

Easily colonise hospital furniture/bathrooms/bed linen and medical devices, e.g. ECG machines, thermometers.

Treatment antibiotics
Intrinsically resistant to many antimicrobials.
Be guided by microbiological advice.★★
Options include:
High-dose ampicillin with high-dose gentamicin if deep-seated infection (beware resistance to aminoglycosides).★★
Quinupristin/dalfopristin (<4% resistance) + doxycycline/rifampicin for bacteraemias, intra-abdominal infections, endocarditis, skin, meningitis and previous treatment failure.
Linezolid – excellent activity against most isolates.★★
Chloramphenicol – useful but risks bone marrow suppression.
Nitrofurantoin – particularly in urinary tract infections.

### References
Lim S, Webb SAR. Nosocomial bacterial infections in intensive care units: organisms and mechanisms of antibiotic resistance. *Anaesthesia* 2005; **60**: 887–902.

## Question 11

A woman who is 36 weeks pregnant and from out of area presents at 4 a.m. to delivery suite complaining of low abdominal pain and vaginal bleeding for 4 hours. She also reports being told she has a 'low-lying placenta'. The obstetric registrar on call asks for your help.
a) Describe your initial assessment of the patient. (30%)
b) Draw a table displaying the severity of the blood loss and common physiological variables. (20%)
The obstetrician tells you that there are signs of fetal distress and that they would like to proceed to delivery by caesarean section.
c) Describe your anaesthetic management of this case. (40%)

### Additional Notes
The advantage of a clinical question like this is that it is easy to think about what you see and do in your day-to-day practice. You are unlikely to be short on inspiration here. Equally, a question like this is a challenge as there is a lot of information to get down. Stick to time and write in notes form. Our full answer here would not be achievable in 15 minutes. Look at the points we have highlighted as essential or desirable and make sure you would have put those down.

### Answer
a) Clinical evaluation of patient in the form of full anaesthetic history paying particular attention to:
Degree of blood loss.★
Cardiorespiratory status especially symptoms of shock,★ significant anaemia and specific questions about airway.
Progress of current pregnancy.★
Previous LSCS (increased risk of placenta accreta).★
Previous blood transfusions.
Drugs, especially anti-platelet therapy and allergies.★
Past medical history.
Family history.
Past anaesthetics.

On examination:

    Careful evaluation of airway.★★

    Vital signs, including pulse rate★★ and character, capillary return,★ skin colour and temperature, blood pressure★★ and oxygen saturations.★★

    In fit, young patients, hypotension is a pre-terminal sign.★★

    Make estimation of degree of haemorrhage.★

    Record weight.

Laboratory tests:

    FBC.★★

    Coagulation screen.★★

    X match★★ 4–8 units★ red cells along with appropriate volumes of FFP and platelets. If clinical suspicion of major haemorrhage use bedside haemoglobin estimation (e.g. Haemacue®).★

Repeated measurement of observations and ongoing assessment of blood loss, i.e. number of pads, haemoglobin.★

b)  See Table 2.

Table 2. *Classification of haemorrhage*

|  |  | Class★ I | Class II | Class III | Class IV |
|---|---|---|---|---|---|
| Blood loss★★ | Percentage★ | <15 | 15–30 | 30–40 | >40 |
|  | Volume★ (ml) | 750 | 750–1500 | 1500–2000 | >2000 |
| Blood pressure★★ | Systolic | Unchanged★ | Normal★ | Reduced★ | Very low★ |
|  | Diastolic | Unchanged★ | Raised | Reduced | Very low/ unrecordable |
| Pulse rate (bpm)★★ |  | <100★ | >100★ | >120 | >140 |
| Capillary refill time★★ |  | Normal★ | Slow (>2 s)★ | Slow (>2 s) | Undetectable★ |
| Respiratory rate★★ |  | 14–20★ | 20–30★ | 30–40 | >40 |
| Urine output (ml/hr)★★ |  | >30★ | 20–30 | 10–20★ | Negligible★ |
| Mental status★ |  | Slightly anxious★ | Mildly anxious | Anxious/ confused★ | Confused/ lethargic★ |

c)  Consent for general anaesthesia and blood transfusion.★

    Call for senior help.★

    Alert haematologist and portering service.★

    Antacid prophylaxis.★

    Two large-bore cannulae.★

    Blood in theatre★ (O negative, or type-specific if not time for fully matched).★

    Full monitoring as per AAGBI guidelines.★

    Measure arterial blood gases★ and urine output.★

    Consider invasive monitoring★ and arm out on board.

    Rapid infuser primed and near by.

    Position supine with left tilt.★

    Pre-oxygenate for >3min.★

    Rapid sequence induction★ of general anaesthesia and tracheal intubation, confirmation of tube placement by clinical means and by measurement of expired $CO_2$.★

    Maintenance of anaesthesia with a volatile agent ensuring adequate depth of anaesthesia, and non-depolarising muscle relaxation.

    Opioid analgesia after delivery of the baby.★

    No more than 5 units of syntocinon given slowly after delivery of baby.★

    Rigorous attention to blood loss and replacement of volume★ with warmed★ fluids.

    Transfuse as dictated by clinical estimation of loss in relation to starting haemoglobin.★

    Repeated bedside haemoglobin estimations to guide transfusion requirement.★

Check for and correct any dilutional coagulopathy or disseminated intravascular coagulopathy with factors +/ – platelets.★★
Don't wait for coagulation studies to give FFP or cryoprecipitate if massive bleeding or transfusion continues.★
Higher risk of atonic lower segment of uterus with ongoing bleeding. May require further uterotonics including syntocinon infusion, misoprostol, ergometrine and caboprost intramuscularly or intramyometrially.
Severe ongoing haemorrhage may require bimanual pressure, 'B-Lynch' brace suture, hysterectomy, balloon catheters in the iliac arteries and/or recombinant factor VII.

### References
Cooper GM, McClure JH. Anaesthesia chapter from Saving Mothers' Lives; reviewing maternal deaths to make pregnancy safer. *BJA* 2008; **100**: 17–22.
Banks A, Norris A. Massive haemorrhage in pregnancy. *Contin Educ Anaesth Crit Care Pain* 2005; **5**: 195–8.

## Question 12

a) How would you identify a patient at risk of postoperative nausea and vomiting (PONV)? (40%)
b) What preventive measures do you take to reduce the chance of PONV? (50%)

### Additional Notes
The second part is a good example of a question that needs to be read carefully. Note that the question does not say after general anaesthesia. It only says postoperative. It is therefore important that non-GA options are discussed.

### Answer
a) In a recent study, postoperative nausea and vomiting (PONV) was the most common complaint following day case anaesthesia. In general, anti-emetics produce a 25% relative risk reduction in PONV. It is important to be able to assess whether a patient is at high risk of PONV to determine whether administration of an anti-emetic as prophylaxis is worthwhile.
The following factors put patients at higher risk of PONV:
Patient factors
   A history of previous PONV★★
   A history of motion sickness★★
   Non-smoker★★
   Female gender★★
   Pregnancy★
   Obesity
   Young and middle-aged adults

Anaesthetic factors
   Prolonged fasting★★
   Gastric insufflation
   The choice of inhalational agent.★ There is a higher incidence than with TIVA★
   More modern inhalational agents produce less PONV than the older agents
   The choice of intravenous agent. There is a higher incidence with etomidate and ketamine
   Nitrous oxide use★★
   Opioid analgesic use★★
   Inadequate analgesia

Anticholinesterase drugs✶
Hypotension✶✶
Hypoxia✶
Intravascular volume depletion✶

Surgical factors
Laparoscopic procedures✶
ENT operations✶
Abdominal procedures✶
Ophthalmic surgery, especially squint procedures✶
Orchidopexy
Hysterectomy✶

b) The following preventive measures should be taken to reduce the chance of PONV:
General measures
Regional anaesthesia (may avoid PONV if hypotension avoided and there is no need for supplemental opioids)✶
Maintain good hydration✶
Avoid hypoxia
Avoid hypotension✶
Avoid gastric insufflation✶
Avoid excessive pharyngeal stimulation, e.g. suctioning
Ensure good analgesia
Use TIVA if possible (propofol is antiemetic)✶
Avoid nitrous oxide✶
Minimise opioid use✶

Antiemetics
Use must be guided by risk stratification.✶
Choice of anti-emetic is mainly driven by side effect profile and cost.✶ No single agent has been found to perform much better than any other.✶ All will produce about a 25% relative risk reduction.✶ Addition of a second agent will add a further 25% reduction to the remaining at-risk group.
Dexamethasone suggested as first line. This should be given well before the end of surgery.✶
5HT3 receptor antagonists reserved for previous severe PONV✶ or as rescue therapy.✶
Cyclizine is a cheap anti-emetic that has a favourable side-effect profile.✶ It may produce tachyarrhythmias in some patients.✶

## Reference

Apfel CC, Korttila K, Abdalla M, Kerger H, Turan A, Vedder I, et al. A factorial trial of six interventions for the prevention of postoperative nausea and vomiting. *N Engl J Med* 2004; **350(24)**: 2441–51.

# Paper 5

Below are the model answers for this paper. ✶✶ indicates essential information, ✶ indicates desirable information and unstarred text is supplementary information. As a guide, an answer with all the essential information and some desirable information would score 50% of the available points.

## Question 1

a) What are the difficulties encountered when managing acute pain in a patient with pre-existing opioid dependence? (40%)
b) How can optimum analgesia be provided for these patients? (50%)

### Answer
a) Opioid dependency may be due to therapeutic or recreational use. ✶
Pain is under-estimated and under-treated. ✶✶
Opioid-dependent patients are often hyperalgesic. ✶
They suffer anxiety ✶✶ about attending for painful procedures as they fear being under-analgesed ✶ or having withdrawal enforced upon them. ✶
If recreational, they may be in an opioid-addiction programme. ✶
Patients on methadone are a particular challenge as they may be 'opioid-tolerant' and 'pain-intolerant'. ✶
Methadone is not given parenterally, so for surgery following which enteral medication cannot be administered the patient will need to be switched to a different opioid to avoid an 'opioid debt'. ✶
Drug interactions occur with methadone. Sedatives increase methadone's depressant effects, and drugs affecting cytochrome P450 will also affect its activity (e.g. discontinuing carbamazepine will put the patient at risk of methadone accumulation).
If the patient is a dependent recreational 'user' with an active habit, difficulties may include:
  Problems with venous access ✶
  An increased risk of psychiatric illness ✶
  Behavioural problems ✶
  Co-morbidity
  The use of other recreational drugs, alcohol and cigarettes ✶

Due to the nature of the problem there is little high-grade evidence.

b) Optimum acute pain management for opioid-dependent patients may include:

Maintaining pre-existing requirements.★★ This could be done with transdermal patches or implantable pumps. It may be as simple as making sure all the patient's normal drugs are written up and administered.★

Preoperative discussion and formulation of a pain-management plan may go a long way to allaying anxiety.★

Giving additional analgesia,★ ideally multimodal,★ with short-acting opioids,★ local anaesthetics,★ ketamine, clonidine, NSAIDs★ and paracetamol.★ Care should be taken if planning to increase a methadone dose to provide additional analgesia as accumulation toxicity is a risk.

If opioids are required and the dose is rising, rather than unsuccessfully increasing the dose, try rotating the type of opioid.★

PCA with higher bolus and shorter lock-out interval is another alternative solution.★★

Ideally avoiding exposing previously addicted patients to opioids. If not possible, opioid therapy should be prescribed.★

If a patient on a methadone program is off methadone for more than 5 days, you should liaise with the patient's drug-treatment centre regarding a re-introduction programme.★

Under no circumstances should analgesia be withheld for fear of the patient becoming addicted/re-addicted.★★

### References

Mehta V, Langford RM. Acute pain management for opioid dependent patients. *Anaesthesia* 2006; **61**: 269–76.

Peng PW, Tumber PS, Gourlay D. Review article: perioperative pain management of patients on methadone therapy. *Can J Anaesth* 2005; **52**: 513–23.

## Question 2

a) Illustrate the anatomy of the circle of Willis. (50%)
b) Describe its physiological importance and the reasons for potential failure of this system. (40%)

### Additional Notes

This question has not been asked before. Cerebral circulatory physiology appears in the primary exam and so should not be new, but the anatomy is often forgotten and is less familiar to most candidates.

# Answer

a) See Figure 12.

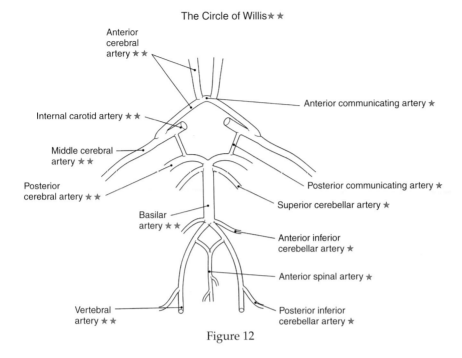

Figure 12

b) Blood enters the circle of Willis from three independent feeding vessels: the basilar artery and the left and right internal carotid arteries.★★

Blood is then distributed to the cerebral arteries (anterior, middle and posterior) and the cerebellar arteries (superior and inferior) via the circle of Willis, facilitating cerebral and cerebellar perfusion.★★

Importance:

Should perfusion from any of the feeding vessels reduce (e.g. internal carotid atheromatous disease), the circle will maintain perfusion to the brain.★★

This occurs as blood from the unaffected feeding vessels continues to contribute to circular perfusion, allowing delivery of blood to all cerebral vessels.★

Thus the circle of Willis provides a safety mechanism, ensuring the preservation of cerebral perfusion in the event of a decrement of flow in one of the main arteries to the brain.★★

This physiological system may fail due to:

Physiological

Flow in the basilar artery is usually insufficient to compensate for bilateral internal carotid occlusion.★★

The cerebellar arteries are relatively proximal to the circle and may be poorly perfused should flow in the basilar or vertebral arteries decrease. This leaves the posterior circulation unprotected by the circle of Willis.★

Congenital

Congenital anatomical abnormalities. The true circle is only seen in 34.5% of patients.★★

Acquired interruption in flow
  From outside the vessel – external compression from mass effect, e.g. tumour, haematoma, abscess.★★
  From the vessel wall itself, e.g. mechanical trauma, subarachnoid haemorrhage, vasculitis.★★
  From within the lumen of the vessel, e.g. atheroma, embolic or thrombotic disease, vasospasm.★★
  Run-off – an intact circle of Willis cannot be assumed to deliver adequate cerebral perfusion as this also requires good run-off from the distal vasculature.★★ This importance is seen clinically in cerebral infarcts affecting watershed areas of the brain.
Pressure
  Although blood may flow in the circle, an adequate cerebral perfusion pressure (CPP) may not be achieved.★★
  Importantly CPP=MAP–ICP–CVP.★

### References

Bergman RA, Afifi AK, Miyauchi R. Illustrated encyclopedia of human anatomic variation: Opus II: cardiovascular system. Circle of Willis, usual and unusual. http://www.anatomyatlases.org/AnatomicVariants/Cardiovascular/Images0200/0291.shtml. (Accessed on 6 August 2008.)
Erdmann A. The brain. In: *Concise anatomy for anaesthesia*. Cambridge. Cambridge University Press. 2007; 42–3.

## Question 3

a) Plastic surgeons often get concerned when performing a free flap operation that the flap may become ischaemic. How might this ischaemia occur? (40%)
b) How, as an anaesthetist, can one ensure that a free flap has the best chance of maintaining adequate perfusion in the intraoperative period? (50%)

### Additional Notes

Anaesthesia for free flap surgery is a big topic so one needs to be precise and concise when answering this one. Unfortunately writing 'I would give them a really good quality anaesthetic like I do for all my patients', though correct, does not score many marks!

### Answer

a) A free flap may be under threat from a number of different mechanisms:
  Primary flap ischaemia★★
    Due to cessation of blood flow to the free flap★
  Ischaemia/reperfusion injury★
    Due to accumulation and then release of inflammatory mediators when blood flow is re-established★
  Secondary ischaemia★★
    Flaps affected by this run into problems with intravascular thrombosis and interstitial oedema★

  Following all surgery under general anaesthesia there are a number of potentially deleterious ways in which blood flow is affected:
    Increased platelet adhesion and aggregation★
    Increased blood viscosity★
    Increased coagulability★
    Impaired fibrinolysis
    Impaired red cell deformability

Combining the above with long surgery time,✷ the potential for large fluid shifts and heat loss✷✷ one can see why anaesthesia for free flap surgery is potentially difficult.

b)  Anaesthetic conduct intraoperatively:
  Maintain high cardiac output✷
  Maintain adequate blood pressure✷✷
  Avoid vasoconstricting agents where possible✷
  Maintain normothermia, with the patient arriving comfortably warm in the anaesthetic room and staying so throughout the perioperative period✷✷
  Institute peripheral AND core temperature monitoring looking for divergent trends. The early use of warming devices✷
  Maintain high urine output✷
  Ensure good analgesia✷
  Monitor haematocrit (viscosity is closely related to haematocrit (Hct) and rises dramatically when Hct is >40% so aim for Hct of 30–35% maximum)✷
  Monitor flow in flap directly (e.g. with Doppler)✷
  Ensure correct venous thrombosis prophylaxis is prescribed and given✷
  Maintain normocapnia to reduce hypocapnic vasoconstriction and hypercapnic sympathetic stimulation✷
  Meticulous attention paid to positioning due to length of surgery✷

  Contentious issues:
  Regional blockade (balance between reduced sympathetic tone, increasing vaso-dilatation against the potential for hypotension)✷
  Crystalloid versus colloid fluid replacement (as always! Probably a mixture of both is the best)
  Dextran administration (theoretically reduces platelet adhesiveness and factor VIII concentration)

### References
Pinnock C, Lin T and Smith T. *Fundamentals of anaesthesia*, 2nd edition. Greenwich Medical Media. 2002; 777–80.
Quinlan J. Anaesthesia for reconstructive free flap surgery. *Anaesth Intensive Care Med* 2006; **7(1):** 31–5.

## Question 4

A 36-year-old woman who has Graves disease presents to the Emergency Department with a cold, pulseless arm of sudden onset. Over the last 3 months she has lost 12 pounds, and developed a hoarse voice. Examination is remarkable for a fine tremor and an obvious goitre. Observations: HR 118/min (irregularly irregular), BP 143/92, temp 37.8°C
  The vascular surgeons wish to perform a CT angiogram and get her to theatre as soon as possible.
a)  How would you evaluate her airway preoperatively? (30%)
b)  What are the specific risks associated with anaesthetising a patient with hyper-thyroidism? (30%)
c)  What drugs would you use to treat her hyperthyroidism? Give a brief description of how each drug exerts its effect? (30%)

### Additional Notes
To ensure nothing is missed in a long clinical question such as this, underline the key words in the question and ask yourself 'What are the major problems in this case?' Here, the major issues at hand are:

Potential airway difficulties
Clinically significant hyperthyroidism
Urgency of the situation (vascular compromise)
Overall perioperative mortality increased

## Answer

a) The candidate should make it clear that, despite the degree of urgency, full assessment of the airway should take place in this patient before surgery.
Six per cent of tracheal intubations for thyroid surgery are difficult.

History
  Positional dyspnoea★★
  Stridor★★
  Dyspnoea on exertion★
  Cough – dry/irritant★
  Hoarseness★
  'Gripping'/constricting feeling in throat
  Dysphagia

Examination
  Routine assessment of airway★★
    Mallampati, jaw protrusion, neck movement, thyromental distance
  Thyroid gland★
    Size
    Texture
    Evidence of retrosternal extension – can you feel below gland?
    Tracheal deviation
  Signs of respiratory distress★★
    Stridor
    Tachypnoea
    Hypoxia
    Recession/obstructive breathing pattern★

Investigations
CXR★
    PA and lateral thoracic inlet views looking for deviated/compressed trachea
    Nasendoscopy – performed urgently by ENT★★
    CT neck/chest – at time of CT angiogram★★
    Arterial blood gases – if any evidence of respiratory distress★
    Pulmonary function tests are not indicated in this setting as will not affect management of patient and will only waste time.

b) Potentially poor pre-morbid state:★
    Malnourished
    Dehydrated
    Associated medical problems – Graves can be associated with:
    Pernicious anaemia
    Diabetes Type 1
    Autoimmune adrenal insufficiency
    SLE
    Medications
    Thioamides (carbimazole/methimazole/propylthiouracil) can cause agranulocytosis, thrombocytopaenia, deranged LFTs.
    Steroids produce long-term complications.

Intraoperatively
  Airway difficulties★★
    Failure to intubate (subglottic compression)
    Loss of airway
    Surgical airway very difficult
  Arrhythmias★★
  CCF★
  Increased sensitivity to catecholamines
  Myocardial ischaemia/infarction★
  Thyroid storm – mortality 20%★★
  High insensible fluid losses★
  Awareness (increased MAC)
  Corneal damage (proptosis)
  Hypercapnia

Postoperatively
  Thyroid storm (can occur pre-, intra- or postoperatively)
  Airway compromise – vocal cord palsy in this patient★

c) (Drug doses would not be expected.)
  Treatment of hyperthyroidism is achieved in four ways:
  Inhibitors of hormone synthesis★★
    Propylthiouracil★★
    Carbimazole★★
    Methimazole

  Inhibitors of hormone release★★
    Potassium iodide/Lugol's iodine – traditionally also used preoperatively to
    reduce vascularity of gland, although not used as much today because gland is
    usually removed in entirety★
    Lithium – second line (narrow therapeutic window)

  Reducing peripheral conversion of T3–T4
    Steroids★★
    Dexamethasone
    Methylprednisone
    Beta blockers – especially propranolol★★

  Reducing the effects of T4
    Benzodiazepines
    Beta blockers★★
      Propranolol – most commonly used
      Esmolol infusion has been described
      Atenolol
      Metoprolol

# Question 5

You are asked to anaesthetise a 32-year-old male for incision and drainage of a groin abscess. He is known to be HIV-positive. Outline the features of your preoperative clinical assessment of this patient that specifically relate to HIV. (90%)

## Additional Notes

Twenty to twenty-five per cent of HIV-positive patients will require surgery at some stage. Patients are often very knowledgeable about their illness/test results/history and this should be utilised. There are likely to be associated complex psychosocial issues. A full history, examination, and ordering appropriate investigations are expected. The candidate will also be expected to identify that this patient may be an IV drug user.

## Answer

Problems specific to this case include:

Chronic poor health
immunosuppressed (may not display signs of sepsis)★★
malnourished★

May be acutely unwell
septic★
dehydrated/hypovolaemic

More likely to be an intravenous drug user★★
Risk of innoculation – universal precautions★★

Old notes should be obtained, examined and a full history taken.
Full anaesthetic history★★
Time since diagnosis★
Previous hospital admissions★
AIDS-defining illnesses, such as:
Candidiasis
Kaposi's sarcoma
Lymphoma
PCP
TB

Drug therapy★★
Antiretrovirals can cause
P450 induction (protease inhibitors)
P450 inhibition (reverse transcriptase inhibitors)
Lactic acidosis
Hepatic steatosis
Cotrimoxazole – suggests patient in more advanced stages of HIV★

Recreational drugs★★
what taken? (especially heroin)
when last taken?
frequency of use
on methadone?★★
Obtain an estimate of amount of opioid taken and therefore required to treat pain and prevent withdrawal.
Other blood-borne viruses – hepatitis B/C★
Last CD4 count

Systems enquiry (looking for evidence of):
RS:
Infection especially PCP (dyspnoea, night sweats, weight loss)★★
TB contacts/travel to high-risk areas★

CVS:
50% of HIV patients have abnormal echocardiographs
Endocarditis (especially in IVDU)★
Pericardial effusion (25%)★
Myocarditis

GIT:
  Diarrhoea (often infective – has implications for nursing)✶
  Candidiasis✶
  Kaposi's sarcoma

CNS:
  Neuropathy
  Dementia

Haem:
  Marrow suppression

Examination
CVS looking for
  Pericardial effusion (25% of HIV-positive patients)
  Murmurs – endocarditis✶
  LVF
  Signs of myocarditis
  Signs suggesting infective endocarditis✶

RS looking for
  Clubbing✶
  Signs of respiratory distress and failure✶

Signs of sepsis/shock✶✶
Venous access/veins✶✶
Hydration status✶✶
Pallor
Teeth – may be carious
Oral candidiasis – possibility of oesophageal/systemic involvement

Investigations
Blood tests✶✶
  FBC✶✶ including CD4 count
  U&E✶✶
  LFTs✶
  ABG if indicated (hypoxic/unwell/dehydrated/septic)✶
  Group and save/cross match depending on Hb
ECG✶
  Left ventricular hypertrophy
  Pericardial effusion
CXR✶✶
  Looking for signs of infection/TB/hilar adenopathy✶
ECHO – if indicated by history✶

## Question 6

a) What are the consequences of intraoperative hypothermia? (40%)
b) Briefly outline the mechanisms by which heat is lost in the anaesthetised patient. (25%)
c) By what means may intraoperative heat loss be minimised? (25%)

### Additional Notes

With the recent publication of NICE guidelines, inadvertent intraoperative hypothermia has become a hot topic. This subject needs to be known intimately for the SAQs and the vivas.

## Answer

a) Hypothermia is defined as a core temperature <36°C.✶✶
   Effects:
   Cardiovascular
      Reduced cardiac output (reduced 30% at 30°C).✶
      J waves on ECG at 30°C.
      Bradycardia followed by ventricular arrhythmias (30°C).✶
      Vasoconstriction.✶
      Increased haematocrit.

   Respiratory
      Apnoea (<24°C).
      Reduced tissue oxygen delivery because of reduced cardiac output,
   vasoconstriction, increased viscosity and shift of the oxyhaemoglobin
   dissociation curve.
      Initially increased oxygen consumption (34°C) followed by reduced oxygen
   demand and $CO_2$ production.
      Shivering on emergence causes increased oxygen demand (500%) at a time when
   the patient is less able to match supply. This may lead to myocardial ischaemia.✶✶

   Neurological
      Heightening of painful sensations
      Confusion (<35°C).✶
      Unconsciousness (30°C).
      Reduced requirement for volatile anaesthetic agents (reduced MAC).✶

   Metabolic/drugs
      Metabolic rate decreases by about 6% per 1°C fall in core temperature.
      Prolongation of neuromuscular blockade and other drug actions.✶
      Impaired coagulation.✶
      Respiratory and metabolic acidosis.
      Reduced GFR.
      Diuresis with reduced ability to reabsorb sodium and water.

   Surgical outcome
      Impaired immunity with increased postoperative infection rates and impaired
   wound-healing.✶
      May prolong hospital stay.

b) Mechanisms by which heat can be lost include:

   Radiation:✶
      50% or more. This is the transfer of heat to a cooler object; this can be an external
   object or internal.

   Convection:✶
      Up to 30%. Air next to body warmed by conduction and carried away
   in convection currents. Increased if large surfaces are exposed to convection
   currents or increased air movement.

   Evaporation:✶
      20–25%. As moisture evaporates from skin or any tissue surface it loses latent heat
   of vaporisation, causing the body to cool. Accelerated if large moist surface
   open to air.✶

   Conduction:✶
      Minor, usually 3–5%. Increased importance if patient lying directly on efficient
   conductor.

Respiration:✱
   10%. Losses due to evaporation in the humidification of inspired air and in its heating to body temperature.

Anaesthesia:✱
   Alters central thermoregulation✱ (hypothalamus), causing vasodilatation, which will increase radiation.

c) Heat loss may be minimised by taking steps to combat the above processes.

   Radiation: ensure patient not in contact with cold air✱ and receives warmed intravenous fluids.✱
   Convection: minimise surface area exposed to room temperature air, especially under laminar flow.✱
   Evaporation: cover open body cavities as much as possible if long periods when no surgery taking place.✱ Replace saturated drapes when possible.✱ If emergency surgery ensure patient stripped of wet clothes as soon as possible and dried.✱
   Conduction: ensure patient not in contact with cold thermal conductor, i.e. insulating mattress on table.✱
   Respiration: use of HME-type device on breathing system to warm and humidify inspired gases✱. $CO_2$ absorber in circle system also warms and humidifies gases in the system.
   Anaesthesia: awareness that active steps must be taken to preserve core temperature in anaesthetised patient.✱

## Reference
NICE Guideline CG65 at http://www.nice.org.uk/Guidance/CG65 (Accessed 30 December 2008.)

## Question 7

a) How should a patient be correctly monitored at induction and during maintenance of general anaesthesia for a high saphenous ligation, strip and avulsions? (50%)
b) What may cause inaccuracies when measuring oxygen saturation using a pulse oximeter? (40%)

## Additional Notes
This feels a bit like a Primary FRCA question, but, with a recent Association pamphlet published on this important topic, the examiner would be looking for a high level of accurate content.

## Answer
a) Core standards of monitoring are essential.✱

   Induction and maintenance:
   Essential:
      Pulse oximeter✱✱
      NIBP✱✱
      ECG✱✱
      Airway gases: $O_2$,✱✱ $CO_2$,✱✱, vapour✱✱
      Airway pressure✱✱

   Available:
      Stethoscope✱✱
      Temperature✱✱
      Nerve stimulator (if NMB drugs used)✱✱

An anaesthetist must be present throughout the anaesthetic. ∗
Appropriate alarm limits with enabled audible alarms. ∗
Anaesthetist to check all equipment before use. ∗ Must be familiar with equipment and had induction in more complex equipment.
Must keep a record. ∗ Electronic records recommended. HR, BP and $SaO_2$ every 5 minutes ∗ or more frequently if unstable.
Handover time and details recorded on chart. ∗
Oxygen analyser with audible alarm continuously monitoring delivered gas is essential. ∗ Vapour analyser essential whenever a vapour is used. ∗∗
If IPPV, airway pressure alarms with appropriate high and low limits are essential. ∗∗
Additional monitoring may be required. Brain function monitoring not routinely indicated.
If an essential monitor is not functional, must be documented.
If cannot be used at induction, e.g. uncooperative confused patient, attach as soon as possible and record in notes.

b) Inaccuracies when using a pulse oximeter may be due to:

Sited on a poorly perfused area ∗∗ due to vasoconstriction ∗ (hypotension, ∗ hypothermia, ∗ hypovolaemia, ∗ heart failure ∗) or peripheral vascular disease. ∗
Venous congestion, ∗ e.g. severe tricuspid regurgitation.
Nail varnish and false nails may produce artificially low readings. ∗
Carboxyhaemoglobin will tend to produce over-reading.
Methaemaglobin will tend to make the oximeter trend towards a score of 85%.
Surgical use of methylene blue may produce inaccuracies.
May underestimate in patients with sickle cell disease. If signal strong, not usually clinically relevant.
Bright lights may interfere with readings. ∗
Shivering or tremor. ∗
Occasionally, diathermy may cause interference with pulse oximetry readings.
Low saturations will be measured less accurately than those above 70%.
Faulty or poorly calibrated equipment.
Time lag. The oximeter reading may lag behind the true value by up to 60 seconds.

### References

AAGBI. Recommendations for standards of monitoring during anaesthesia and recovery. 2007; 4th edn. Online at http://www.aagbi.org/publications/guidelines/docs/standardsofmonitoring07.pdf (Accessed 3 January 2009.)

## Question 8

a) What are the potential advantages and disadvantages of a critical care outreach team? (45%)
b) In 2007 the National Institute for Clinical Excellence (NICE) published a document 'Acutely Ill Patients in Hospital'. Outline its main recommendations. (45%)

### Additional Notes

Outreach is a topic that is high up the critical care agenda at the moment. There have been numerous national bodies advocating the development of outreach services in hospitals and with a limited healthcare budget early identification and treatment of high-risk patients would seem sensible both in terms of improving outcome but also for the efficiency of healthcare provision in this 'expensive' patient group. However, outreach is controversial, a seemingly commonsense idea that has not been backed by consistent outcome data, hence this lends itself well to an advantages/disadvantages question. The second part of the question tests topical knowledge. Knowing what the big healthcare organisations are up to is important in SAQ prediction.

## Answer

a) An outreach service should have three main goals:

To identify patients at risk of critical illness and then either prevent admission or facilitate early admission to a critical care unit.★★
To provide follow-up for patients leaving a critical care unit.★★
To share critical care skills with ward staff.★

Advantages of critical care outreach
Care can come to the patient irrespective of location within the hospital★
Ward staff feel better supported★
Cost (early identification of at-risk patients may prevent high-cost critical care unit admission and reduce patient length of stay)★★
Early identification of patients for whom critical care admission is inappropriate★★
Reduction in unexpected admissions to critical care, allowing better resource planning★★
Sharing of critical care skills through observation and training★
Potential for audit and research★
Reduction in readmissions following discharge from critical care by outreach team follow-up★★

Disadvantages of critical care outreach
Deskilling of ward team★★
Cost (staffing costs to run system) ★★
Little evidence of benefit★
No accurate data on who should be part of the team hence inconsistency of team make-up nationally.

b) This document was written in an attempt to improve the identification and subsequent management of the acutely unwell or deteriorating patient.★ It stresses the importance of making sure staff are adequately trained to fulfil the recommendations.★
Recommendations include:

All patients should have physiological observations recorded on admission and a plan set out for how often (minimum 12 hourly) after that.★★
Physiological 'track and trigger' systems should be implemented so there is a method of identifying a deteriorating patient and a threshold system for initiating a graded response.★★
This graded response should be divided into three levels (low, medium and high).★ What this graded response should be should be decided at a local level.
The decision to admit the patient to critical care should involve both the critical care and ward consultants.★
Transfer between or out of critical care should not take place between 22.00hrs and 07.00hrs if at all possible.★★
There should be a formal handover of the patient (both into and out of the critical care unit) and the ongoing care of the patient should be on a shared care basis.★★

**References**
National Institute for Clinical Excellence (NICE) 2007: Acutely ill patients in hospital. Online at http://www.nice.org.uk/nicemedia/pdf/CG50FullGuidance.pdf (Accessed on 31 December 2008.)
DeVita M, Bellomo R, Hillman K, et al. Findings of the First Consensus Conference on Medical Emergency Teams. *Crit Care Med* 2006; **34(9):** 2463–78.

## Question 9

a) What are the risk factors for development of post-dural-puncture headache (PDPH)? (40%)
   A woman who received an epidural as part of her pain relief during labour develops a headache 6 hours post-delivery, after the epidural catheter has been removed.
b) List the differential diagnoses of her headache. (10%)
c) If this turns out to be a PDPH, outline your subsequent management. (40%)

**Additional Notes**
There is quite a lot in this question so when it says list then list! The first part to this question can be divided into patient and operator factors. Remember not all PDPH headaches occur in pregnancy. The second is reasonably straightforward but again it is important to think outside the loop on this one. Management of PDPH should be core knowledge.

**Answer**
a) Risk factors for PDPH are:
   Patient factors
       Female sex (women twice as likely as men to develop PDPH).✶
       Obesity (increased risk of accidental dural puncture).
       Age between 18 and 40 years old.
       History of headache prior to dural puncture.
       Previous history of PDPH.✶
       Of interest some meta-analyses have failed to show that pregnancy per se is an independent risk factor.

   Operator factors
       Needle shape and size.✶✶ Dural puncture with large,✶✶ cutting✶✶ needles causes the highest incidence of PDPH (70–90% of all parturients after accidental dural puncture with a 16 gauge Tuohy needle compared to less than 1% with 25–27 gauge pencil point needles).
       Inexperience of operator.✶✶
       Epidural insertion technique.✶ Perpendicular orientation of the bevel of a spinal or epidural needle is associated with a reduction in PDP.

b) Differential diagnoses for post-partum headache:
       PDPH.✶✶
       Tension, stress, fatigue, depression, idiopathic.✶✶
       Pre-eclampsia.✶✶
       Infection, e.g. meningitis, sinusitis.✶✶
       Migraine.✶
       Raised intracranial pressure secondary to tumour, haemorrhage, venous thrombosis or benign intracranial hypertension.✶

c) Treatment options are divided into symptom alleviation✶✶ while the dural hole heals and/or an attempt to seal the hole.✶✶

Symptomatic treatment options include:

Simple analgesics.★★

Ensure adequate fluid intake.★★

Caffeine either as tablets, coffee or carbonated drinks.★ Aim for 600mg/day in divided doses.

Anecdotal evidence exists for sumatriptan (serotonin receptor agonist) and ACTH; the latter by increasing the concentration of beta-endorphin and therefore intravascular volume.

Epidural blood patch:

This is now the definitive treatment of choice★★ and tends to be performed early in the PDPH history. Two separate mechanisms of action:

Compression of the dural sac raises intracranial pressure, often causing immediate cessation of the headache.★

Sealing of the dural leak by the blood clot, so preventing further CSF loss.★

Repeat blood patching may be necessary★ and serious complications are rare★.

## References

Yentis S, May A, Malhotra S, Bogod D, editors. *Analgesia, anaesthesia and pregnancy: a practical guide*, 2nd edition. Cambridge University Press. 2007; 111–16.

Turnball D, Shepherd D. Post-dural puncture headache: pathogenesis, prevention and treatment. *Br J Anaesth* 2003; **91(5):** 718–29.

## Question 10

a) List the potential advantages of percutaneous tracheostomy over prolonged endo-tracheal intubation in a patient ventilated on critical care. (50%)
b) How would you assess whether a patient is safe to have their tracheostomy removed (decannulated)? (40%)

## Additional Notes

This question has some black and white parts to the answer but also some grey. There are a number of ongoing trials looking at percutaneous tracheostomies within critical care patients and it may be worth a one-liner stating this at the start of your answer. For part (b), make sure you think about a safe and structured approach.

## Answer

a) Percutaneous tracheostomy

Reduces the need for ongoing sedation compared with endotracheal intubation.★★

Allows continuing respiratory support with a patient fully awake.★★

Improves the ability to maintain oral hygiene.★

Reduces the incidence of lip, intra-oral (including teeth) and glottic trauma due to the endotracheal tube and the method used to secure tube position.★

Is less likely to be pulled out, so reducing the risk of accidental extubation.★

Is less likely to be pushed down too far, reducing the risk of one-lung ventilation.★

May produce a reduction in long-term vocal cord problems.★

Reduces dead space and the work of breathing. This may augment weaning from ventilatory support.★

Reduces the incidence of tube obstruction and allows the patient to speak with an appropriate device attached.★

May produce a lower incidence of ventilator-associated pneumonia and there is better secretion removal with suctioning.★

Allows easier administration of aerosol-type medication (e.g. nebulised agents).

Probably reduces length of stay within a critical care unit.

Reduces dependency level during that stay.

b) Before considering decannulation there are a number of checks one can go through:

Has the reason for needing a tracheostomy in the first place resolved?✲✲ The decision to remove a tracheostomy from a patient with fully resolved upper airway obstruction is very different to tracheostomy removal in a patient with resolving Guillain Barre.

Has the need for mechanical ventilation gone and is there no anticipated future need (e.g. a return to theatre for surgery)?✲✲

Is the patient haemodynamically stable?✲

Has their swallow been assessed as adequate (e.g. by a speech and language assessment)?✲

Does the patient have a suitable conscious level?✲

Can the patient cough adequately to clear secretions?✲

A patient-generated maximum expiratory pressure of >40cmH$_2$O may be useful.

### References

Christopher K. Tracheostomy decannulation. *Respir Care* 2005; **50(4):** 538–41.

Rumbak M, Newton M, Truncale T, Schwartz S, Adams J, Hazard P. A prospective randomised study comparing percutaneous dilatational tracheotomy to prolonged translaryngeal intubation (delayed tracheotomy) in critically ill medical patients. *Crit Care Medicine* 2004; **32:** 1689–94.

## Question 11

a) What characteristics set remifentanil apart from other opioid analgesics and why? (40%)

b) What problems are common to all sedative agents within a critical care setting? (20%)

c) What are the potential advantages of switching from a hypnotic-based sedative regime to an analgesic-based sedation regime using remifentanil? (30%)

### Additional Notes

Remifentanil is no longer the 'new kid on the block' so it seems somewhat surprising that, to date, there has been no mention of it in the SAQ part of the exam. It must be coming up soon!

There has been recent focus on sedation in critical care in part due to a push from the manufacturers of remifentanil to encourage its use within critical care. A consensus document on sedation strategies in critical care is expected shortly.

In part (c), bear in mind these are potential advantages so you have a bit more artistic license in your answer.

### Answer

a) Remifentanil is a synthetic phenylpiperidine derivative (like fentanyl, pethidine and alfentanil) that is a selective μ-opioid agonist.✲✲

Uniquely amongst opioid drugs it is metabolised by blood and tissue esterases✲ (and not plasma cholinesterase as is often mistakenly thought).

Its metabolite has no opioid activity but does accumulate in renal impairment, unlike remifentanil itself✲

It has the smallest volume of distribution of all the opiates.

As a result of its mechanism of metabolism, remifentanil is unique in its context-sensitive half time (CSHT).✲✲

This is defined as the time for the plasma concentration to decline by half, after the termination of an infusion designed to maintain a constant plasma concentration.

The 'context' refers to the duration of the infusion. The CSHT for remifentanil is approximately 3 minutes* (it does increase slightly in the elderly) and is independent of the duration of the infusion**.

b) Problems common to all sedative agents include:

Accumulation with prolonged infusion so delaying weaning from mechanical ventilation.**

Detrimental circulatory effects leading to increased need for vasoactive medication.*

Increased VQ mismatch leading to the need for increased ventilatory support.*

Tolerance during drug administration and withdrawal problems on cessation.*

Lack of REM sleep during sedation, which is an important cause of critical care psychosis.*

Reduction in intestinal motility.*

Immune system depression.

c) Sedation in critical care carries a morbidity and mortality.

Daily sedation holds have been shown to reduce both the duration of mechanical ventilation and the length of stay in the critical care unit.**

Finding a sedative agent (or combination of agents) that allows the patient to be comfortable, pain free, calm and co-operative, yet does not mean they are asleep all the time, can be problematic. * There are a number of potential advantages in changing the focus of sedation in critical care from a hypnotic-based one to an analgesic-based one using remifentanil. These include:

Reduction in propofol use.

Increase in patient comfort.*

Less dose adjustment needed in patients with hepatic and/or renal impairment.*

Patient is more awake.*

Easier dose titration.*

Allows better interaction with nurses and relatives.

Possible cost benefits (cost of remifentanil versus reduction in time on mechanical ventilation + reduction in hypnotic agents + shorter stay in critical care).*

## References

The Intensive Care Society sedation guideline. Online at www.ics.ac.uk/icmprof/downloads/sedation.pdf (Accessed 24 December 2008.)

Muellejans B, López A, Cross M, Bonome C, Morrison L, Kirkham A. Remifentanil versus fentanyl for analgesia based sedation to provide patient comfort in the intensive care unit: a randomised double-blind controlled trial. *Critical Care.* Online at http://ccforum.com/content/8/1/R1 (Accessed 24 December 2008.)

## Question 12

What are the special considerations when anaesthetising a patient with probable variant CJD requiring gamma-nailing of a fractured femur? (90%)

## Answer

Creutzfeldt-Jakob disease (CJD) is a transmissible spongiform encephalopathy (aka prion disease).

It is a fatal neurodegenerative disease. Prions are found in brain cord and eye.*

In 1996 a new form was described: variant CJD (vCJD).*

The average age of patients diagnosed with vCJD is 29.

By 2003, 130 definite or probable cases had been diagnosed in the UK.

A substantial epidemic now looks unlikely (death rate peaked in 2000).

Uniquely, in vCJD, prions are also found in lympho-reticular tissue.✷

Prions are small enough to reside in crypts on stainless steel.✷ They are not deactivated by traditional methods.✷✷

Patients with probable or known vCJD may present for anaesthesia for MRI, tonsillar biopsy, PEG, or as emergencies.✷✷

Arrangements for such a case require substantial logistical planning and need as much notice as possible.✷

> The hospital's communicable disease officer will need to be contacted for local policy.
> It is helpful to ascertain the certainty of diagnosis. Cases are defined as either:
>> Definite vCJD diagnosed by brain biopsy
>> Probable vCJD diagnosed by tonsillar biopsy or clinical features +MRI +EEG
>> Possible vCJD diagnosed by clinical features and EEG✷

> The certainty of diagnosis will determine how to organise disposal equipment.✷
> At the preoperative visit the following problems may be present:
>> Aggression✷
>> Drooling (consider antisialogogue)
>> Dysphagia
>> Poor communication✷
>> Anxious relatives✷

The following precautions should be taken:
> The operating theatre should be stripped down and minimum staff present.✷
> Warning signs on doors.✷
> All staff in double gloves, masks, goggles, aprons and liquid-repellent gowns.✷
> Sharps into bin for immediate incineration.
> Single-use equipment where possible.✷
> Keep everything simple.
> Use portable suction which follows patient to ward.✷
> Send all used equipment for incineration at end of procedure.✷
> Try to avoid diathermy as the smoke plume may contain prions.✷
> Ventilator dedicated to that patient. Stripped of disposables and cleaned at the end.✷
> If the patient has a potentially difficult airway, a fibreoptic endoscope is available from CJD Surveillance Unit.
> If the diagnosis is only suspected, re-usable equipment should be washed and dried then sealed in a cytotoxic container and bag, then stored until the diagnosis is made.✷

## Reference

Farling P, Smith G. Anaesthesia for patients with Creutzfeldt-Jakob disease. A practical guide. *Anaesthesia* 2003; **58**: 627–29.

# Paper 6

Below are the model answers for this paper. ✷✷ indicates essential information, ✷ indicates desirable information and unstarred text is supplementary information. As a guide, an answer with all the essential information and some desirable information would score 50% of the available points.

## Question 1

a) Describe the anatomy of the coeliac plexus. (40%)
b) What are the indications for coeliac plexus blockade? (10%)
c) How is blockade of the coeliac plexus performed? (40%)

### Additional Notes
At first sight, this question may terrify you. Chronic pain is appearing more and more in the exam and there are only a handful of nerve blocks used in chronic pain which are fair to ask in the exam. Unfortunately, this is one of them, so it is worth learning well.

### Answer
a) The coeliac plexus is a mixed autonomic plexus responsible for the innervation of abdominal viscera and vasculature. ✷✷
   There are two coeliac plexi found to the left and right of the coeliac trunk at its origin from the aorta at the level of L1. ✷✷
   The relations of the plexi are:

   Superior – crura of the diaphragm ✷✷
   Inferior – coeliac trunk and its branches (hepatic, splenic and left gastric arteries) ✷✷
   Anterior – pancreas ✷✷
   Posterior – abdominal aorta ✷✷

The plexus receives preganglionic sympathetic fibres from the greater, lesser and lowest splanchnic nerves, originating from T5–T9, T10–T11 and T12 respectively. ✷
It also receives a branch from the posterior vagal trunk, derived mainly from the right vagus nerve. ✷
Postganglionic fibres emerge to innervate the vasculature, musculature and secretory cells of the stomach, small and large bowel as far distally as two-thirds of the way along the transverse colon, the pancreas, liver and gallbladder, spleen and in part the supra-renal glands.

b) Indications are:
1. Relief of pain (especially malignant in nature) from intra-abdominal non-pelvic organs, e.g. carcinoma of the stomach and pancreas, acute and chronic pancreatitis.★★
2. Intra-abdominal analgesia during surgery.
May be diagnostic or therapeutic.★

c) Performing the block:

Patients must be fully consented and have intravenous access in situ.★★
The block should be performed in a clean, well-lit environment with resuscitation drugs and equipment and fully trained assistance available.★★
Patients may be in the lateral or prone position.★
Sterile technique: prep and drape.★★
Locate the needle insertion site 5–10cm from the midline, level with the spinous process of L1.★★
Insert a 10cm needle at 45° to the skin. Direct the needle medially and slightly cranially to pass over the transverse process so that the needle tip lies anterior to the upper part of the body of L1.★★
Initially perform a test injection of 15–25ml 1% prilocaine or 1% lidocaine with adrenaline after prior aspiration.★★
If beneficial, a second injection of 25ml 50% alcohol may be carried out at a later date to provide analgesia of several months duration.★
The needle must be flushed prior to withdrawal to prevent alcohol deposition along the needle tract.★

**Reference**
Moore KL, Dalley AF. The abdomen. In: *Clinicallly orientated anatomy*. Lippincott Williams & Wilkins. 1999; 230–48.

## Question 2

A 72-year-old male patient is undergoing an open reduction and internal fixation of the right ankle under general anaesthesia following a fall 1 day previously. Thirty minutes after the start of surgery, you notice ST elevation on the ECG.
a) What is your immediate management? (45%)
b) How would you proceed in light of persisting ST elevation once the wound is closed? (45%)

**Additional Notes**
The structuring of this answer will differentiate the strong from the weak candidates. It is essential to avoid a flurry of perfectly valid but disorganised suggestions which may leave the examiner confused and concerned about your ability to prioritise. It is likely to further impress the examiner if you can relate your therapeutic decisions to the first principles which underlie them.

**Answer**
a) 1. Call for help and stop operating immediately.★★
2. Assess using an ABCDE approach:
   A – Ensure a patent airway and the delivery of 100% oxygen through patent anaesthetic equipment.★★
   B – Ensure adequate bilateral ventilation – auscultate, ensure $SaO_2$>95%, $ETCO_2$ 4.8–6.0kPa and airway pressures are <30cm$H_2$O.★★
   Do an arterial blood gas.★
   C – Assess the pulse, blood pressure, peripheral perfusion, blood loss; do a 12-lead ECG and send blood (FBC, G&S, clotting, U&E, glucose and magnesium).★★

If ST changes confirmed on the 12-lead ECG:

Decrease myocardial oxygen demand
> Ensure adequate depth of anaesthesia. Consider fentanyl 100μg bolus.✶✶
> If tachycardia, reduce rate with β-blocker, e.g. esmolol 0.5mg/kg loading then infusion 50–200μg/kg/min.✶
> Treat arrhythmias as appropriate.✶
> In the absence of hypotension deflate tourniquet to reduce afterload; surgeon to obtain haemostasis.
> Reduce preload with sublingual GTN then GTN infusion 50mg in 50ml; 3ml/hr titrated to effect.✶✶ Consider putting slightly head-up.✶

Increase myocardial oxygen supply
> Give blood to ensure Hb >10g/dL and fluid to ensure adequate perfusion pressure.✶✶ Consider CVP guidance.
> If perfusion pressure remains poor give vasopressor (e.g. metaraminol 0.5mg); if contractility poor consider inotrope (e.g. dobutamine 5–10μg/kg/min).✶✶
> Give aspirin 300mg sublingually or rectally and enoxaparin 1mg/kg subcutaneously.✶✶ Consider 20mg simvastatin orally at the first available opportunity.✶

b) The aim must be to redress the balance of oxygen supply and demand.

Awakening the patient will greatly increase oxygen demand and should not be attempted.
Thrombolysis is contraindicated given the surgical insult.

> Maintain anaesthesia.✶✶
> Call for urgent cardiological help with view to urgent percutaneous intervention (PCI).✶✶ Prepare to transfer the anaesthetised patient to the catheter lab safely using portable monitoring equipment and drugs and trained assistance.✶
> Pass an NG tube and give Clopidogrel 300mg.✶
> Liaise with cardiologists re Abciximab.
> Maintain the rate pressure product (heart rate × systolic pressure) <12 000 using the techniques described above.✶
> Ensure adequate oxygen delivery using the techniques described above.
> Ensure normal plasma electrolyte, glucose and haemoglobin levels. An insulin sliding scale with glucose and potassium (GKI) may be required.
> Liaise with the ICU for postoperative care.✶✶

## Reference
Allman KG, McIndoe AK, Wilson IH. Intraoperative myocardial ischaemia. In: *Emergencies in anaesthesia*, 1st edition. Oxford. Oxford University Press. 2005; 30–1.

## Question 3

What investigations should be performed on a patient suspected to have had an anaphylactic reaction under an anaesthetic you administered? (90%)

### Answer
Immediate investigations:✶
The key to diagnosing anaphylaxis is the appropriate sampling to test mast cell tryptase.✶✶
Blood (5–10ml) venesected and sent in a plain tube.✶✶
Samples should be taken immediately,✶ at 1 hour,✶ at 6 – 24 hours✶ or post-mortem and the times the samples were drawn must be written on the sample tubes.✶
The correct drawing of samples should be recorded in the patient's notes.

The peak tryptase level occurs 1 hour after degranulation but may be earlier in severe cases.

Serum is separated and stored at 4°C (refrigerator) if the investigation will occur within 24 hours.✶ If the investigation is likely to be longer, the sample should be stored at −20°C.

Elevated levels indicate mast cell degranulation and define the event as anaphylactic or anaphylactoid.✶

A negative test does not rule out anaphylaxis.✶ It is possible to have mild anaphylaxis without a raised tryptase.

Having determined whether or not anaphylaxis occurs, later investigations are required to determine the causative agent.✶

Later investigations:✶
Investigation into causation must not interfere with the immediate treatment of the patient, and can usually occur at a later date.✶

If anaphylaxis is suspected, the patient should be fully investigated.✶

The anaesthetic team (consultant, or trainee and consultant) are responsible for making sure investigation occurs and the results are followed up.✶

The patient should be referred to an allergist (preferably Regional Allergy Centre).✶

Investigation is predominantly scrutiny of clinical management, looking through the history with particular reference to timing and the agents to which the patient was exposed.✶ As much useful clinical information as possible should be sent such as notes, including drug and anaesthetic charts and a detailed clinical description of the event, including timing.

Tryptase analysis may be required if the tryptase was borderline.

At least 4 weeks after the reaction, the patient should have skin tests.✶

Skin prick tests will usually be performed first.✶ These detect IgE.

Intradermal skin tests may be required. These are more sensitive and invasive.

IgE serum antibodies can be measured for some drugs. The only anaesthetic drug for which this is used is suxamethonium. This test is very sensitive and expensive.

If latex allergy is suspected the patient may require skin testing, or measurement of IgE by radioallergosorbent testing (RAST) or fluoro-immunoassay (CAP©).✶

### Reference

AAGBI. Suspected anaphylactic reactions associated with anaesthesia. 2003. 2nd edn. Online at http://www.aagbi.org/publications/guidelines/docs/anaphylaxis03.pdf (Accessed 30 December 2008.)

## Question 4

A 46-year-old woman is listed for a laparoscopic cholecystectomy as a day case. She weighs 113kilos and is 150cm in height. What anaesthetic challenges does this case present? (90%)

### Additional Notes

Obesity is a major global health problem. NICE have recently looked at obesity and made recommendations. These two factors mean that the College is likely to be regularly visiting this topic for questions. Anaesthetising the obese patient is core knowledge for the Final FRCA. This answer is over an achievable word count in a 15-minute essay. A good candidate would be looking to cover all the major points in this answer.

### Answer

Laparoscopic cholecystectomy:

Laparoscopic surgery presents its own set of challenges. Most of these relate to the pneumoperitoneum cuffing the intra-abdominal large vessels✶ and placing restriction on respiratory excursion.✶ These will be exacerbated in the obese patient. Other factors such as working in the dark or the increased technical difficulty and therefore duration of the surgery should be taken into account.

Day case surgery:

Obesity is only a relative contraindication to day case surgery.✶ Many units are happy to perform simple operations on patients with a body mass index (BMI) of 40 if they are otherwise fit and well. Laparoscopic cholecystectomy is a procedure that centres are performing on selected patients on a day case basis. The combination of a complex operation and a Class III obese patient would make this case inadvisable to be carried out as a day case.✶✶

Obesity:

BMI 50✶✶ Class III obesity defined if BMI >40.✶
This degree of obesity presents many challenges:

Airway:

Increased soft tissue in the pharynx making it difficult to maintain airway for bag/mask ventilation.✶
Decreased ability to flex head on neck.✶
Laryngoscopy may be difficult.✶
Increased likelihood of hiatus hernia reflux disease necessitating rapid sequence induction.✶✶

Breathing:

Reduced/absent FRC when supine making pre-oxygenation difficult and desaturation more rapid, therefore RSI less safe.✶
Fat deposition on chest and on/in abdomen results in high inflation pressures for IPPV.✶✶
Hypercapnia and hypoxia more likely.
Slow equilibration with volatile anaesthetics.
May have obstructive sleep apnoea (OSA) (5%)✶ and therefore be very sensitive to respiratory depression with anaesthetic agents and opioids. This may make successful extubation difficult and may require period of CPAP postoperatively, perhaps in an HDU environment.✶
More prone to postoperative desaturation even in absence of OSA.
In extreme cases may have Pickwickian syndrome (obesity, somnolence, polycythaemia, pulmonary hypertension and right ventricular failure).

Circulation:

Vascular access may be difficult.✶
Monitoring of ECG and NIBP is more challenging due to body habitus. May require an arterial line for reliable BP monitoring.✶
More prone to hypertensive disease (50–60%).
Increased risk of coronary artery disease and cardiomyopathy.
Increased blood volume and cardiac work.
Increased incidence of type 2 diabetes mellitus (×5) with associated increased risk of macro- and microvascular disease, including ischaemic heart disease (more prone to 'silent' ischaemia and infarction), renovascular disease and diabetic nephropathy, cerebrovascular disease and peripheral vascular disease.✶
More prone to cellular hypoxia.
Increased risk (×2) of deep vein thrombosis.✶

Neuro:

If diabetic, autonomic neuropathy makes BP more labile and delays gastric emptying, increasing likelihood of reflux and aspiration.

Drugs:

> Increased volume of distribution for fat-soluble drugs*. In particular, may take a long time to breathe off volatile agents.
> Difficulty estimating ideal body weight for drugs limited to central compartment.*

Miscellaneous:

> Regional techniques more challenging.*
> Manual handling issues for whole theatre team.*
> Will require an appropriate table and bed.*

### Reference

AAGBI guideline. The perioperative management of the morbidly obese patient. June 2007. Online at http://www.aagbi.org/publications/guidelines/docs/Obesity07.pdf (Accessed 30 December 2008.)

## Question 5

An otherwise fit and well 52-year-old woman presents for surgery for acoustic neuroma. The surgeon informs you that this is a technically difficult case which he anticipates taking 10 to 12 hours. What are the problems and what specific measures would you take when anaesthetising such a long operation? (90%)

### Additional Notes

Although this answer is over on word count, most of the content could be included in 15 minutes if the answer was written in notes form or a series of expanded bullet points.

### Answer

Airway and ventilation:

> All the usual measures for an intracranial neurosurgical operation are required in this case. The patient will require intubation and ventilation. This is particularly important as the case is at risk of atelectasis.* A small amount of PEEP may be useful.*
> An HMEF should be used to reduce heat and water loss, and to stop airway secretions drying out.*
> Cuff size changes should be anticipated, checked and corrected.* Pilot balloon needs to be accessible.
> The choice of oxygen concentration is controversial.* Some groups maintain that high oxygen concentration improves wound healing and outcome. Others are concerned that it will produce small airway collapse. Oxygen with air mix giving an $FiO_2$ of 0.6 should satisfy both arguments.*
> Venting the breathing system is advocated by some for long cases using minimal flow anaesthesia through a circle system. The accumulation of gases such as methane has never been shown to be clinically significant. It is possible theoretically for the circuit to accumulate carbon monoxide if the patient is a very heavy smoker. If this is the case, flows of >1 l/min should be used.

Monitoring:

> Pulse oximeter positioned carefully and moved every 2 hours.*
> An arterial line is mandatory** for BP monitoring, and blood sampling for blood gases, blood sugar and Hb measurement.
> Long cases are at increased risk of thromboembolic disease and will require pneumatic calf compression devices.*
> A central venous catheter may be useful to guide fluid replacement.

Blood loss may be underestimated.⋆ A small amount of haemorrhage over a long time may become significant.

A urinary catheter with hourly measuring bag is required⋆⋆ to avoid soiling⋆ and allow hourly urine output measurement.⋆⋆

Pressure care:

Great care needs to be taken with positioning and pressure-point care.⋆⋆ This is important at the beginning of the case when the patient is initially set up on the table, but must also continue throughout the case.⋆

Vulnerable areas such as the elbows and heels need extra attention, with care taken to ensure they are well padded and protected.

The patient should be placed on a soft mattress,⋆ with a crease-free sheet.⋆

No stress on limb joints should be the aim when positioning.⋆ Care should be taken to position the knees in a slight flexed position rather than full extension.

Particular care with how monitoring lines and other equipment run.⋆ Try to avoid contact pressure with the patient by careful positioning or padding where necessary. Do as much of a head-to-toe check as possible, every 2 hours.⋆⋆ Also re-check every time the operating table is moved.⋆

The eyes need to be protected⋆⋆ to avoid any foreign body entering the eye, or pressure placed on the globe. This should be checked every 2 hours.

Drugs:

Second or more doses of antibiotics should be given at appropriate intervals.⋆

Choice of anaesthetic agents to avoid accumulation and allow rapid emergence is important.⋆⋆ Remifentanil and desflurane would be an acceptable choice that will permit rapid postoperative assessment.⋆

Temperature:

Inadvertent hypothermia or hyperthermia is a potential problem.⋆ Temperature should be monitored and the patient kept normothermic. Don't overheat.

Logistics and teamwork:

During long cases there is a genuine risk of losing concentration.⋆⋆ It may be helpful to have two anaesthetists working on this case, ensuring adequate breaks and cross-checking each other's work.⋆ Verbal communication between the anaesthetists involved needs to be excellent and an accurate anaesthetic record must be kept meticulously.⋆

It is also likely that the theatre personnel will change throughout the case. Making sure everyone entering the team understands what is happening is important.⋆

## References

Allman KG, Wilson IH. *Long operations. Oxford handbook of anaesthesia*. Oxford University Press. 2001: 582–3.

Boisson-Bertrand D, Laxenaire MC, Mertes PM. Recovery after prolonged anaesthesia for acoustic neuroma surgery: desflurane versus isoflurane. *Anaesth Intensive Care* 2006; **34**: 338–42.

## Question 6

a) The oxygen saturation in the left ventricle of a foetus is 65%. List the physiological mechanisms that allow the foetus to tolerate this degree of relative hypoxaemia. (40%)

b) What pharmacokinetic differences between adults and neonates are relevant to anaesthesia? (50%)

## Additional Notes

This question requires an extension of the knowledge of the foetal circulation, testing whether you have simply rote-learned the facts or have stopped to question them. Consider answering any question on pharmacokinetics using the structure outlined below in order to trigger ideas and avoid missing important points. Giving examples where possible improves the quality of an answer.

## Answer

a) Anatomical

The crista terminalis ensures oxygenated (67%) IVC blood is preferentially directed to the left heart via the foramen ovale, deoxygenated (40–50%) SVC blood being preferentially directed to the right heart.✶

Biventricular ejection results in well-oxygenated blood (65%) perfusing the heart and brain because the deoxygenated blood from the ductus arteriosus enters the aorta distal to the left subclavian.✶✶

This ensures the vital organs receive the highest possible $PO_2$.✶✶

Physiological

High placental blood flow for rapid reoxygenation.✶✶

HbF has low levels of 2,3-DPG, increasing the affinity of haemoglobin for oxygen and shifting the oxyhaemoglobin dissociation curve to the left.✶✶

HbF therefore has p50 = 20mmHg compared with adult maternal HbA of 30mmHg, ensuring a steep gradient for placental transfer of oxygen.✶✶

The foetus has a very high oxygen delivery rate $(DO_2)$✶✶ as both the cardiac output (Q=300–400ml/kg per min) and the haemoglobin concentration ([Hb]=17–18g/dL) are high and:

$DO_2 = Q ([Hb] \times SaO_2 \times 1.39) + (0.003 \times PO_2)$

b) Pharmacokinetic differences

Absorption

GI tract

Decreased gastric acid secretion with higher pH and slower gastric emptying times (premature children) can lead to unreliable GI absorption.✶✶

Rectal

Variable venous drainage. Drug may enter portal circulation and undergo first-pass metabolism.

Percutaneous

Thin, well-perfused skin increases absorption of drug.✶

Intranasal

No first-pass metabolism. Bioavailability of midazolam = 57% intranasal vs 30% oral.

Intramuscular

Poor muscle bulk and unpredictable blood flow produces unpredictable absorption.✶

Distribution

Higher cardiac output delivers drugs to effector site more rapidly.✶✶

Less protein binding = more free drug.✶

Due to a combination of decreased protein quantity (neonatal albumin = 35g/L, adult = 45g/L) and decreased protein quality (fetal albumin has lower affinity for drug).

Increased total body water and ECF and decreased total body fat. ↑$V_d$ for water soluble drugs (e.g. non-depolarising muscle relaxants) and ↓$V_d$ for fat-soluble drugs.✶✶

Metabolism
  Phase 1. P450 oxidation (immature), reduction (variable), hydrolysis (fully mature).✶✶
  Phase 2. Conjugation immature, e.g. glucuronyltransferase deficient until 6 months.✶
  Affected by hepatic blood flow, which can fall in illness.

Elimination
  Reduced renal blood flow (5% of cardiac output) and reduced renal perfusion pressure lengthens half-life of renally eliminated drugs (e.g. ampicillin).✶✶
  Limited ability to excrete fluid load.
  Limited concentrating ability risks dehydration.✶✶
  50% reduction in pseudocholinesterase.✶
  More rapid Hoffman degradation✶

## Question 7

a) What markings are present on the valve block and body of an oxygen cylinder? State where these markings are (cylinder body or valve block). (50%)
b) For transfer of a 70kg intubated and fully ventilated patient on a journey anticipated to take 120 minutes, calculate how much oxygen you would take to ensure safe transfer. Show your calculations and assumptions. Give your answer in litres and number of 'E'-sized cylinders. (40%)

### Additional Notes

This is a 'you either know it or you don't' question. It is fair game in the exam and an example of something we use day in day out that may just need looking at a bit more closely as the exam approaches. As practice for the exam, sit in front of an anaesthetic machine complete with circuit attached and make sure you can describe and explain all the component parts from where the pipes leave the ceiling to the mask attached to the end of the catheter mount.

### Answer

On the valve block (the bit that screws into the open end of the cylinder):
  Pin index system if cylinder is to be screwed into an anaesthetic machine.✶✶ 2 and 5 position for oxygen, 3 and 5 for nitrous oxide, 1 and 5 for air and 7 for Entonox.✶
  Serial number that is unique to each cylinder.✶
  Tare weight.✶ This is the mass of the empty cylinder AND valve block.
  Symbol of the contained gas.✶✶
  Pressure of the last hydraulic test.✶

There may also be one or more variably coloured plastic disks around the valve block. These disks are put on when a cylinder is tested.
On the cylinder itself:
  Colour coding.✶✶ For oxygen, black body and white shoulders.✶✶ (Make sure you know the rest including the rare ones. I got asked about xenon in my viva!)
  Name and symbol of the gas.✶
  Volume and pressure of the contained gas.✶
  A label giving details about flammability and risk of explosions,✶✶ the owner of the cylinder and who manufactures the oxygen contained within.

b) The AAGBI publication 'Recommendations for the safe transfer of patients with brain injury' recommends that for a transfer you should carry a minimum of

1 hour or twice the anticipated journey length of oxygen, whichever is the greater volume.★★ Therefore in this situation:

Assuming the patient is ventilated on 100 % $O_2$★
Minute volume = tidal volume × respiratory rate★★
Tidal volume = approximately 10ml/kg.★★ Respiratory rate estimated at 10/min.★★
Therefore, minute volume = 10ml/kg × 10 = 7000ml or 7 litres★
Number of minutes = 120 × 2 (twice anticipated journey length) = 240min★
Therefore $O_2$ required = 240 × 7 = 1680 litres.
$O_2$ cylinder capacities are as follows:

| | | |
|---|---|---|
| C size | 170 | litres |
| D size | 340 | litres |
| E size | 680 | litres★★ |
| F size | 1360 | litres |

So you will need 3 E cylinders minimum for a safe transfer.★

### References

Pinnock C, Lin T, Smith T. Fundamentals of anaesthesia, 2nd edition. *Greenwich Medical Media*. 2002; 9–10.

Advanced Life Support Group. Oxygen therapy and monitoring. *Safe transfer and retrieval: the practical approach. 2nd edition. Blackwell BMJ Books*. 2006; 59–78.

Recommendations for the safe transfer of patients with brain injury 2006. Online at www. aagbi.org/publications/guidelines/docs/braininjury.pdf (Accessed 3 January 2009.)

## Question 8

a) What are the symptoms and signs of a right-sided pleural effusion? (30%)
b) State how pleural effusions can be classified and give examples of each. (20%)
c) What tests need to be performed on a sample of pleural fluid to identify the nature of the effusion? (40%)

### Additional Notes

This is a test of your clinical skills and your knowledge base. Show the examiner that you have both by including additional information such as Light's criteria. It is a basic, compact topic so lends itself to the SAQ exam. Be sure to classify your answer well.

### Answer

Defined as fluid between the visceral and parietal pleura.★★

a) Symptoms
    Dyspnoea★★
    Chest discomfort★
    Symptoms related to the underlying disease process – loss of appetite, weight loss, lethargy (malignancy); cough, fever, rigors, night sweats (infection).★★

  Signs detectable on the right:
    Reduced chest expansion.★★
    Stony dullness to percussion.★★
    Reduced tactile vocal fremitus and increased volume of whispering pectoriloquy.★★
    Reduced breath sounds to auscultation.★★
    Displacement of the mediastinum to the left if very large effusion.★

b) Pleural effusions may be classified into transudates and exudates.★★

Transudates
  Raised venous pressure
    Fluid overload★★
    Cardiac failure★★
  Hypoproteinaemia
    Cirrhosis★★
    Nephrotic syndrome★
    Protein-losing enteropathy
    Hypoalbuminaemia★★
  Other
    Hypothyroidism★
    Yellow nail syndrome

Exudates
  Infection
    Pneumonia, empyema, subphrenic abscess★★
  Malignancy
    Primary disease (of lung or pleura) or secondary deposit★★
  Trauma
    Haemothorax, chylothorax, oesophageal perforation★★
  Autoimmune
    RA, SLE, sarcoid★
  Other
    Post-infarction (PE or MI-Dressler's syndrome), pancreatitis★

c) Tests

Inspection of pleural fluid★★
The differentiation of transudate and exudate is based on Light's criteria,★★ such that if ≥ 1 of the following are present, the effusion is an exudate, if none is present the effusion is a transudate:
1. Ratio of pleural fluid protein to serum protein > 0.5.
2. Ratio of pleural fluid LDH to serum LDH > 0.6.
3. Pleural fluid LDH > 2/3 upper limit for serum.

It is therefore imperative to test both blood *and* pleural fluid for:
  Protein
  LDH

Measuring pleural protein alone (<30g/L transudate; >30g/L exudate) is less accurate. Other tests:

Microscopy, culture and sensitivity★★
  Identifies cell types present (neutrophils, red cells, macrophages, etc.) and identifies an infecting micro-organism as well as its sensitivity to antimicrobial therapy.
Additional tests of infection
  Gram stain★★
  ZN stain (for TB)★
  Fungal stain
Glucose★★
  Low in rheumatoid effusion, TB and some empyemas.
pH (normally 7.62)★★
  Low in inflammatory and infiltrative processes (infection, malignancy, oesophageal rupture).

Cholesterol
>    Elevated in chylothorax.
Amylase★
>    Elevated in acute/chronic pancreatitis and oesophageal rupture.

**Reference**
Paramasivam E, Bodenham A. Pleural fluid collections in critically ill patients. *Contin Educ Anaesth Crit Care Pain* 2007; **7**: 10–14.

# Question 9

a) What are the patient risk factors that are known to influence surgical risk? (50%)
b) List the physiological variables required to calculate a P-POSSUM score. (40%)

**Additional Notes**
Preoperative risk assessment is perhaps the hottest topic in anaesthetic practice at the present time. This is linked to the concept that better allocation of resources is possible the earlier that patients are identified as being at the greatest perioperative risk. The POSSUM scale (Physiological and Operative Severity Score for the enUmeration of Mortality and morbidity) is a scoring system that is used to predict risk-adjusted mortality and morbidity rates in a wide variety of surgical procedures. POSSUM is becoming more widely used in the UK as surgical culture moves more towards out-come measures and providing the patient with as much information as possible to make fully informed consent. Furthermore a system that uses risk-adjusted prediction is going to become an essential clinical governance tool.

**Answer**
a) The factors affecting surgical risk clearly vary with the type of surgery the patient is undergoing.★ However, in the huge (87 000+ patient) Veterans Affairs Surgical Risk Study, patients undergoing non-cardiac operations were investigated. This study identified 26 preoperative variables for predicting operative mortality and 28 preoperative variables associated with postoperative morbidity in patients undergoing general surgery. Of these the 10 most significant, when all the different non-cardiac surgical specialities were grouped together, were (in order, most significant first):

>    Serum albumin (low level, associated with poor outcome)★★
>    ASA class.★★ Table 3, adapted from the Veterans Affairs Study data, shows the dramatic increase in mortality for increasing ASA status:

Table 3. *ASA and mortality*

| ASA | Mortality (%) – large bowel obstruction due to colorectal cancer |
|-----|------------------------------------------------------------------|
| I | 2.6 |
| II | 7.6 |
| III | 23.9 |
| IV | 42 |
| V | 66.7 |

>    Emergency CEPOD (Committee of Enquiry into Perioperative Death) class of operation★★
>    The presence of disseminated cancer★★
>    Age★★

The rate of mortality increases almost exponentially with age through most of the adult age range but this tends to slow down at very old ages. A possible explanation for this is the selective survival of healthier individuals to older ages.

DNR status✶

Thrombocytopenia (platelets <150 000/μl)✶

Operative complexity✶

Significant weight loss (>10%)✶

Presence of renal impairment✶

Other risk factors included:

The presence of dyspnoea, ascites, hepatomegaly, ventilator dependence, hyponatraemia, being on haemodialysis, the presence of a tumour involving the nervous system, a high white cell count and hypokalaemia.

b) POSSUM scoring

There are different POSSUM scores that can be used depending on the surgical group being examined. For example, CR-POSSUM is used in patients undergoing colorectal surgery and O-POSSUM is used in patients undergoing oesophagogastric surgery. P-POSSUM can be applied to general surgical patients. It uses 12 physiological parameters and six operative ones.✶

Physiological parameters:

Age✶✶

Cardiac status✶✶

Respiratory status✶✶

ECG✶

Systolic BP✶✶

Pulse rate✶✶

Haemoglobin✶

White cell count✶

Urea✶

Sodium✶

Potassium✶

Glasgow coma score✶✶

Operative parameters:

Operation type (minor, moderate, etc.)

Number of procedures

Operative blood loss

Peritoneal contamination

Malignancy status

CEPOD class

Once the data is put in, a predicted morbidity and mortality is calculated.

**References**

Risk prediction in surgery website. Online at http://www.riskprediction.org.uk (Accessed on 30 December 2008.)

Khuri S, Daley J, Henderson W, *et al*. Risk adjustment of the postoperative mortality rate for the comparative assessment of the quality of surgical care: results of the National Veterans Affairs Surgical Risk Study. *J Am Coll Surg* 1997; **185(4):** 315–27.

## Question 10

a) What is pre-eclampsia and how is it diagnosed? (20%)

b) List the effects of pre-eclampsia on maternal physiology. (30%)

c) Describe the principles of management of a patient with pre-eclampsia, giving examples. (40%)

## Additional Notes

At time of writing, a question on pre-eclampsia has never before been asked in the short answer questions. Given that this represents core knowledge and that pre-eclampsia features in every CEMACH report, it must just be a matter of time before a question on this topic arises.

This question tests both detail and breadth of knowledge on the subject, showing that both sound knowledge and a structured approach in constructing an answer are essential. Be guided by the distribution of marks to ensure your time is appropriately spread and read the question carefully – anaesthetic management is not asked for here and will not score points.

## Answer

a) Pre-eclampsia is defined as gestational proteinuric hypertension developing after 20 weeks gestation.★★
It is associated with new-onset proteinuria, resolving after delivery.

Diagnosis requires:
Pregnancy >20 weeks gestation★★
Hypertension (diastolic BP >90mmHg or a rise of >15mmHg)★★
Proteinuria (>300mg/24 hours)★★
With or without oedema★

b) Physiological effects:

Cardiovascular
↑ SVR.★★
Low or normal plasma volume.★★
↑ myocardial contractility (↑ or normal cardiac output).
Giving ↑ cardiovascular strain and hyperdynamic left ventricle.★

Respiratory
↓ colloid osmotic pressure and damaged vascular endothelium risks pulmonary oedema and ARDS.★★
Particularly evident with inappropriate IVI being compounded post-partum as sequestered tissue water is remobilised.

Renal
Glomerular capillary endotheliosis (capillary endothelial cell engorgement).★
Reversible unless compounded by pre-existing renal disease.
Oliguria and proteinuria.★★
Oedema.★★

Hepatic
Fibrin deposits in sinusoids.
Subcapsular haematoma.
Periportal necrosis (↑ transaminases).
If severe these phenomena may obstruct hepatic blood flow→ liver distension, pain.★★
HELLP (hypertension, elevated liver enzymes, low platelets) with potential hepatic rupture.★★

Haematology
Microangiopathic haemolysis.★
Thrombosis consumes platelets and risks DIC.★★

Neurology

    38% have no symptoms prior to eclampsia.✶

    Hypertensive encephalopathy and cerebral vasospasm.✶

    Thrombosis causes micro-infarctions.

    Cerebral oedema.✶✶

    CVA/subarachnoid bleed.✶✶

c) Management

    Aims:

        Minimise vasospasm

        Improve perfusion of uterus and vital organs

        Assess fetal maturity and timely delivery

        Prevent eclampsia

        BP control

    Magnesium sulphate.✶✶

        4g over 15mins, then 1g/hr for 24hrs then review. Further 2g bolus if eclamptic fit.✶

        Aim for 2–4mmol/L.

    Labetolol (if no asthma)✶✶

        200mg orally repeated in 30min if needed then…

        50mg IV repeated in 5min if needed.

        20mg/hr IV infusion, doubled every 30min to max 160mg/hr.

    Nifedipine (second line or labetolol contraindicated)✶✶

        10mg PO repeated in 30min.

    Hydralazine (third line)✶✶

        5mg IV bolus, infusion 5–15mg/hr.

    Epidural anaesthesia✶

        Adjunct. Ideally platelets $>100\times10^9$/L prior to insertion.

    Avoid ergometrine/syntometrine in third stage.✶✶

    Obtund pressor response to intubation if GA.

        Alfentanil, $MgSO_4$, esmolol, labetolol or lidocaine.✶✶

    Fluid management

        Careful.✶✶ Restrict to 1ml/kg per hr.

        Hourly urine output; tolerate oliguria 0.25ml/kg per hr.✶

        If below this for 4hrs insert central line aiming for CVP 0–5mmHg.✶

        Avoid diclofenac.

    Timely delivery

        Steroids (betamethasone) if gestation <34 weeks.✶✶

        TEDS and clexane post-delivery if platelets >100.✶

## References

Hart E, Coley S. The diagnosis and management of pre-eclampsia. *Contin Educ Anaesth Crit Care Pain* 2003; **3**: 38–42.

Scrutton M, Kinsella M. Severe pre-eclampsia. In: Allman K, McIndoe AK, Wilson IH eds. *Emergencies in anaesthesia*. Oxford. Oxford University Press. 2005; 154–6.

## Question 11

a) What are the indications for inserting a spinal cord stimulator? (50%)

b) What are the complications of this procedure? (40%)

## Answer

a) In 2005, The British Pain Society published the following guidelines for indications for spinal cord stimulator (SCS):

Good indications for SCS (likely to respond):
Neuropathic pain in leg or arm following lumbar or cervical spine surgery (failed back surgery syndrome).★★
Complex regional pain syndrome.★★
Neuropathic pain secondary to peripheral nerve damage.
Pain associated with peripheral vascular disease★★ due to atherosclerosis,★ diabetes,★ Raynaud's,★ Buerger's★ and vasospastic disorders.★
Refractory angina or small vessel vasospastic disease (Syndrome X).★★
Brachial plexopathy★: traumatic (partial, not avulsion), post-irradiation.

Intermediate indications for SCS (may respond):
Amputation pain (stump pain responds better than phantom pain).★
Axial pain following spinal surgery.★
Intercostal neuralgia, e.g. post-thoracotomy or post-herpetic neuralgia.
Pain associated with spinal cord damage.
Other peripheral neuropathic pain syndromes, e.g. following trauma, may respond.

Poor indications for SCS (rarely respond):
Central pain of non-spinal-cord origin.
Spinal cord injury with clinically complete loss of posterior column function.
Perineal, anorectal pain.

Unresponsive to SCS:
Complete cord transection.
Non-ischaemic nociceptive pain.
Nerve root avulsion.

b) Complications of SCS:

Major complications are rare. The following is a list of more common★ or rare and potentially serious★ complications that should be discussed when consenting a patient for SCS:
Dural puncture and CSF leak with possibility of a severe postural headache.★★
Procedural failure.★
Direct nerve damage at insertion.★
Epidural infection★★ or haematoma.★★ Nerve damage from these is reversible. Patients need to be observed post-procedure and have early access to appropriate radiological investigation.
Infection of implanted device.★ Will usually require removal unless superficial.
Equipment failure★ of lead and electrode, battery, pulse generator or telemetry. This may occur immediately or a part may fail after a time. The need for repeat procedures to maintain or repair the device should be explained.★

## References

Spinal cord stimulation for the management of pain: recommendations for best clinical practice. A consensus document prepared on behalf of the British Pain Society in consultation with the Society of British Neurological Surgeons. March 2005. Online at http://www.britishpainsociety.org/book_scs_main.pdf (Accessed 1 January 2009.)
Carter ML. Spinal cord stimulation in chronic pain: A review of the evidence. *Anaesth Intensive Care* 2004; **32**: 11–21.

# Question 12

a)  What devices are available to deliver drugs to a patient transdermally? (20%)
b)  What factors influence the systemic uptake of transdermally applied drugs? (40%)
c)  How can the uptake of transdermally applied drugs be increased? (30%)

## Additional Notes

This question would be difficult to answer if you had not read the corresponding article in the continuing education bulletin that you receive from the College. You should keep abreast of these, especially in the run-up to the exam.

Transdermal drug delivery is a developing science in which there is currently a great deal of interest. Many new devices have recently been released into the marketplace, showing efficacy approximating those of standard PCA regimes.

## Answer

a) Drugs are delivered via a transdermal patch. There are two types:

1.  Reservoir.**
    Drug is held in gel or solution and delivery is controlled by a rate-controlling membrane.*
    This affords tight control of delivery rate, after an initial bolus.
    Damaging the membrane risks sudden overdose.
2.  Matrix.**
    Drug distributed evenly about a polymer matrix, such that half a patch delivers half the hourly dose.*
    The amount of drug held in the matrix and the area of skin contact determine the dose.
    Less risk of accidental overdose and therefore abuse.

b) Systemic uptake is affected by:

Skin
    Variation in thickness of stratum corneum of epidermis**
    Skin hydration**
    Skin disease/injury
    Ethnic differences
    Body temperature and therefore skin perfusion*
    The presence of shunt pathways (e.g. sweat glands) may increase uptake.

Drug/patch
    Rate of drug passing per unit time = $(D \cdot C_0 \cdot K)/h$*
    Where $D$=diffusion coefficient, $C_0$=concentration of drug in patch, $K$=partition coefficient and $h$=thickness of membrane.
    Drugs of low molecular mass (high $D$), high solubility (high $C_0$) and patches affording a high $K$ will permit rapid systemic uptake.**
    Drugs of this nature include fentanyl and GTN.*

c) Drug uptake can be increased by:

Skin
    Abrading the stratum corneum prior to application of patch.**
    Removing skin oils prior to application of patch.**

Drug
    Enhance the drug's solubility by adding ethanol or propylene glycol.

Iontophoresis**
    The application of an electric field to drive charged particles across the skin.

The drug is dissolved in an electrolyte solution and is surrounded by an electrode of the same polarity.

An electrode of opposing polarity is placed elsewhere on the body, completing the circuit.

Application of electromotive force drives the drug into the skin; uncharged molecules are drawn into the skin by a convective action known as electro-osmosis, allowing a bolus function equivalent to that of a PCA.

## References

Chelly JE, Grass J, Houseman TW, *et al*. The safety and efficacy of a fentanyl patient-controlled transdermal system for acute postoperative analgesia: a multicentre placebo controlled trial. *Anaesth Analg* 2004; **98**: 427–33.

Margetts L, Sawyer R. Transdermal drug delivery: principles and opioid therapy. *Contin Educ Anaesth Crit Care Pain* 2007; **7**: 171–6.

# Paper 7

Below are the model answers for this paper.✶✶ indicates essential information,✶ indicates desirable information and unstarred text is supplementary information. As a guide, an answer with all the essential information and some desirable information would score 50% of the available points.

## Question 1

a) How is $CO_2$ transported in arterial and venous blood? (20%)
b) Illustrate graphically how the $CO_2$ content of blood varies with $PaCO_2$. (15%)
c) Why is $CO_2$ transport better in deoxygenated than oxygenated blood? (25%)
d) What does sodalime contain and how does it eliminate $CO_2$ from a circle system? (30%)

### Additional Notes

$CO_2$ carriage is something that can be a bit tricky to get one's head around. A good diagram or two may make life much easier.

### Answer

a) Approximately 50ml of $CO_2$ is carried per 100ml of arterial blood✶ compared to 55 ml per 100ml of venous blood.✶
   $CO_2$ is 20-times more soluble in blood than $O_2$.✶
   $CO_2$ is carried in three main ways✶✶ :

|    |                          | Arterial (%) | Venous (%) |
|----|--------------------------|--------------|------------|
| 1. | Dissolved in blood       | 5            | 10         |
| 2. | As bicarbonate           | 90✶✶         | 60         |
| 3. | As carbamino compounds   | 5            | 30✶        |

$CO_2$ can be carried as bicarbonate shown by the reaction:
$$CO_2 + H_2O \leftrightarrows H_2CO_3 \leftrightarrows H^+ + HCO_3^- ✶$$
This occurs in erythrocytes.

b) See Figure 13.

## Dissociation of carbon dioxide versus oxygen

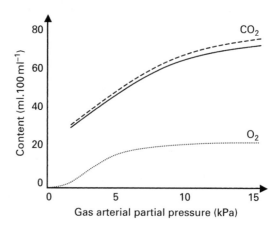

## Carbon dioxide dissociation curves

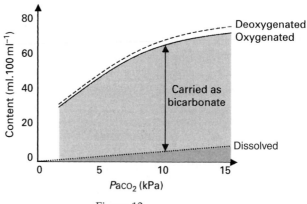

Figure 13

c) The Haldane effect explains how deoxygenated haemoglobin carries more $CO_2$. ✶
   There are two main reasons:
   Deoxyhaemoglobin forms carbamino compounds more readily with $CO_2$ than oxyhaemoglobin✶✶ hence there is more $CO_2$ carried as carbamino compounds in venous blood.
   Deoxyhaemoglobin acts as a buffer for the $H^+$ ions formed✶ thus increasing the amount of $HCO_3^-$ created. So although the percentage of $CO_2$ carried in venous blood as bicarbonate is lower, the actual amount is not. The $HCO_3^-$ created diffuses out of the erythrocyte in exchange for $Cl^-$ ions. This is known as the Hamburger Shift.

d) Sodalime is a granulated compound containing $Ca(OH)_2$✶✶ and $NaOH$.✶✶ It has to have a water content to work effectively✶ and also an indicator✶ (usually by colour change) to show exhaustion. Some sodalimes contain small amounts of potassium hydroxide.✶
   The chemical reactions are as follows:

$$CO_2 + H_2O \rightarrow H_2CO_3$$

$$CO_2 + 2NaOH \rightarrow Na_2CO_3 + 2H_2O + heat\star$$
$$Na_2CO_3 + Ca(OH)_2 \rightarrow 2NaOH + CaCO_3 + heat\star$$

### Reference

Cross M, Plunkett, E. *Physics, pharmacology and physiology for anaesthetists. Key concepts for the FRCA*, 1st edition. Cambridge Medicine. 2007; 137–8.

## Question 2

a) How would you classify recreational drugs? Give three examples in each class. (25%)
b) How would you classify controlled drugs? (15%)
c) What are your responsibilities as an anaesthetist when handling controlled drugs? (50%)

### Answer

a) Recreational drugs are classified under the Misuse of Drugs Act 1971 into three classes (A, B and C).★★ Class A drugs are the group widely thought to be the most harmful.★★ Possession or dealing in Class A drugs generally carries a higher penalty than Class B, which in turn is viewed as a more serious offence than Class C drugs.

   Class A drugs include ecstasy,★ cocaine,★ heroin,★ LSD,★ methadone,★ morphine,★ methylamphetamine★ and injectable forms of class B drugs.

   Class B includes cannabis,★ oral preparations of amphetamines,★ barbiturates, methylphenidate (Ritalin) and codeine.

   Class C includes most benzodiazepines★ and other less harmful drugs of the amphetamine group, gammahydroxybutyrate (GHB), anabolic steroids and ketamine.★

b) Controlled drugs are classified under the Misuse of Drugs Act 1971 into the following groups:
   Schedule 1  No medical use, e.g. LSD.
   Schedule 2  Pharmaceutical opioids★ and amphetamines.
   Schedule 3  Barbiturates.★
   Schedule 4  Benzodiazepines.★
   Schedule 5  Low concentration Schedule 2 drugs.

c) Your responsibilities as an anaesthetist when handling controlled drugs are:
   Sign for drugs used.★★
   Record in notes the amounts used.★★
   Return unopened ampoules.★
   Dispose of any unused controlled drugs that remain in an ampoule or syringe.★
   Do not share ampoules between patients.★
   Store CDs in secure but accessible place.★
   Dispose of CDs appropriately.★
      Local guidelines are required; Department of Health guidelines are due soon. CD ceases to be classified once denatured, dissipated, is not re-usable or has been rendered irretrievable.★ Should be unrecognisable. Empty syringes before discarding.
   For PCA use pre-filled syringes where possible.
   To recognise the changing roles of staff.

### References

AAGBI Guideline. Controlled drugs in perioperative care. (Jan 2006). Online at http://www.aagbi.org/publications/guidelines/docs/controlleddrugs06.pdf (Accessed 3 January 2009.)

The Home Office Drugs Website http://drugs.homeoffice.gov.uk/drugs-laws/misuse-of-drugs-act/ (Accessed 24 December 2008.)

## Question 3

a) Draw a transverse section through the spinal cord at the level of the third cervical vertebra (C3) showing the ascending and descending neural pathways. (50%)
b) Describe the symptoms and signs which may result from:
– a unilateral cord lesion in the thoracic spine at the level of the fourth thoracic vertebra (T4). (20%)
– a complete transverse cord lesion in the thoracic spine at T4. (20%)

### Additional Notes

It is worth spending a bit of time learning the pathways seen in a cross section of the cord. It crops up in vivas as well and if you know it, you can always work out the subsequent answers.

### Answer

a) See Figure 14.

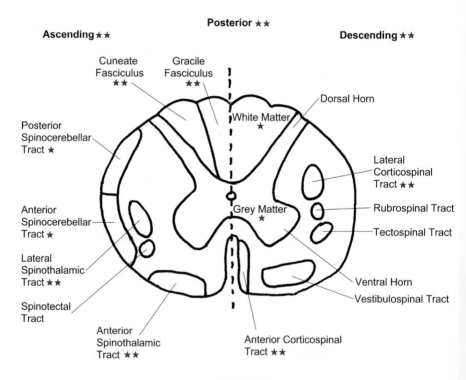

**Transverse Section Through C3 Showing Ascending and Descending Pathways ★★**

Figure 14

b) Unilateral cord lesion
    This is the Brown Sequard syndrome★★★ and will interrupt:

Sensory tracts

The ipsilateral gracile and cuneate fasciculi carrying sensations of proprioception, vibration and discriminative touch.✶✶

The contralateral spinothalamic pathway carrying sensations of temperature, pain and crude touch.✶✶ This will be detectable 2–3 segments below the level of the lesion.

Spinotectal and spinocerebellar tract interruption will accentuate the loss of proprioceptive input and interfere with spinovisual reflexes.✶ This may result in loss of balance, ataxia and intention tremor but compensation may occur from the unaffected hemicord.

Descending tracts

The ipsilateral lateral and anterior corticospinal pathways carrying pyramidal and extrapyramidal fibres respectively. This will result in an ipsilateral loss of motor function and hypertonia with brisk reflexes.✶✶

The ipsilateral rubrospinal, tectospinal and vestibulospinal pathways. The clinical implication of interruption of these pathways cannot be identified given the ipsilateral loss of motor function.✶

Positive ipsilateral babinski sign (upgoing plantar) will be seen, which may be absent in acute injury.✶✶

Complete transverse cord lesion

The clinical picture varies with the time since injury. In the dermatomes and myotomes below the level of injury, the clinical picture is:

Initially:

Bilateral weakness, flaccid paralysis, areflexia and complete sensory loss (light and crude touch, proprioception, pain and temperature).✶✶

Interruption of vascular tone may result in hypotension with warm peripheries below the level of injury (spinal shock).✶✶

Bradycardia is less likely with injury at T4 (seen with injuries above T1), but arrhythmias may be seen.✶

Subsequently:

Spastic paralysis, hyperreflexia with persisting complete sensory and motor loss in the dermatomes and myotomes below the level of injury.✶✶

Weak and ineffective cough with vital capacity only 20% of normal.✶✶

Paralytic ileus.✶

Risk of autonomic dysreflexia.

## References

Kumar P, Clark M. Lower motor neurone (LMN) lesions. In: *Kumar and Clark Clinical Medicine*, 5th edition. W.B. Saunders. 2004; 1148–52.

Yentis SM, Hirsch NP, Smith GB. Spinal cord. In: *Anaesthesia and intensive care A-Z. An encyclopaedia of principles and practice*, 3rd edition. Butterworth-Heinemann. 2005; 483–4.

## Question 4

a) What is the physiological role of magnesium in the body? (30%)
b) List the indications for the use of magnesium as a therapeutic agent. (30%)
c) What are the harmful effects of magnesium therapy which may be seen in the context of anaesthesia? (30%)

## Additional Notes

Magnesium remains a popular topic in anaesthetic exams and a useful drug in clinical practice, but many candidates have difficulty in producing a confident, coherent summary. The only question in the SAQ exam was asked in 2001 shortly after the publication of the BJA CEPD review… so be prepared for further adaptations of this topic in forthcoming exams.

## Answer

a) Physiological role
   Essential co-factor in >300 enzyme systems, especially those:

   Linked with ATP★★
     This makes it essential for the workings of the Na/K ATPase transmembrane pump and therefore for the maintenance of sodium and potassium transmembrane gradients throughout the body.★★
     Intracellular concentrations of calcium and potassium are also regulated by magnesium-dependent ATPases.
   Linked with adenyl cyclase and the generation of cAMP★★
     This impacts on intracellular signalling, most importantly the release and actions of parathyroid hormone, having a pivotal role in calcium homeostasis.★
   Linked with oxidative phosphorylation and glucose metabolism★
     Involved in the production of DNA, RNA and regulation of protein function★
   Calcium and catecholamine antagonist:★★
     Depresses myocardial contractility★
     Anti-arrhythmic properties★★
     Reducing pulmonary and peripheral vascular tone★ and response to vasoconstrictors (but conversely permissive action for adrenaline)
     Dose-dependent pre-synaptic inhibition of ACh release at neuromuscular junction★★
     Also directly depresses neuromuscular excitability and is important for muscular contraction/relaxation★★
     Clotting cascade inhibitor
     Reduces thromboxane synthesis resulting in less platelet aggregation.
     Suppresses epileptic foci and reverses cerebral vasospasm.
     NMDA antagonist so has a role in analgesia★

b) Therapeutic uses
   Replacement of loss, e.g. GI tract losses

   CVS
     Antiarrhythmic (prolongs SA and AV node refractoriness so useful in SVT, VT with prolonged QT interval and digoxin toxicity)★★
     Specifically indicated in torsade de pointes★★
     Prophylactically after cardiopulmonary bypass
     Obtund blood pressure swings in phaeochromocytoma★
   Respiratory/airway
     Acute severe bronchospasm★★
     Obtund the pressor response to laryngoscopy and extubation★
   Other
     Prevention and treatment of eclampsia★★
     Tetanus
     Autonomic hyperreflexia
     Osmotic laxative when administered orally

c) Harmful effects
   Nausea and vomiting★
   Headache★
   Somnolence
   Potentiation of non-depolarising neuromuscular blockade and areflexia★★

Hypotension, exacerbated by agents such as volatiles, induction agents and possibly epidural anaesthesia✶✶
Muscular weakness with potential respiratory embarrassment✶
AV and intraventricular conduction disorders✶
Respiratory and cardiac arrest

### References

Watson VF, Vaughan RS. Magnesium and the anaesthetist. *Contin Educ Anaesth Crit Care Pain* 2001; **1**: 16–20.
Sasada M, Smith S. Magnesium sulphate. In: *Drugs in anaesthesia and intensive care*, 3rd edition. Oxford University Press. 2003; 236–7.

## Question 5

a) Briefly describe how an image is generated by a magnetic resonance imaging (MRI) scanner. (45%)
b) What are the particular difficulties in anaesthetising a patient within an MRI scanner that are different from those in other remote locations? (45%)

### Additional Notes

'Anaesthesia in remote locations' type questions have come up a few times in the past. However, a specific MRI one was last seen 8 years ago so may be due a reappearance. Remember to read the question. If you see the word 'particular', be specific!

### Answer

a) The beauty of MRI is the absence of ionising radiation.✶ The strength of the magnetic field they produce is measured in teslas. Typical medical MRIs produce 1.5 to 3 T. Each tesla is about 30 000 times more powerful than the Earth's magnetic field.
An MRI scanner produces three sorts of magnetic field:
Static, continuous magnetic field
Pulsed radiofrequency fields
Fast switching magnetic fields – called gradient magnetic fields

The principles behind MRI are that the body is composed predominantly of water molecules✶✶ and that each of these contains two protons or hydrogen nuclei.✶✶
In the presence of a static magnetic field the protons in the water molecules align in the direction of the field.✶✶
A second radiofrequency magnetic field is then briefly turned on and the protons absorb some of this energy.✶ When this second field is switched off the protons release this energy and this can be detected by the scanner.✶
By continuously applying additional magnetic fields an image can be built up.
An MRI scan is able to differentiate different tissue types because protons in different tissues return to their equilibrium state at different rates.✶

b) The particular difficulties in anaesthetising a patient within an MRI scanner are:
Access to the patient once in the scanner is extremely difficult due to the tunnel length and diameter.✶✶
MRI scans can be lengthy procedures and the temperature in the scanner is often lower than in an operating theatre, putting the patient at risk of hypothermia.✶
Monitoring has to be MRI-compatible and often gives poor quality readings,✶✶ may be unfamiliar to the anaesthetist✶ and is prone to interference by the magnetic fields,✶✶ in particular the gradient ones.
Acoustic noise.✶✶ The trend towards stronger and faster scanners means that noise within a scanner may increase further. This is a potential hazard for both staff and patients.

Magnetic fields induce eddy currents in electrical conductors (e.g. ECG leads) which may affect electronic equipment.✲

The magnetic field generated attracts ferromagnetic objects, which may become projectiles.✲ Electric motors on syringe drivers may fail✲ and any data stored electronically may be wiped if it gets too close to the magnetic field.✲ Hence scanning 'ITU'-type patients is extremely difficult.

All the hazards of ventilation down long breathing systems✲ should be considered; e.g. ventilator pressure readings at the ventilator end not accurately representing those at the patient end and tidal volume 'dialled up' being considerably less than that delivered due to compression of the gas within the tube.

### References

AAGBI. Provision of Anaesthetic Services in Magnetic Resonance Units. May 2002. Online at http://www.aagbi.org/publications/guidelines/docs/mri02.pdf (Accessed 28 December 2008.)

Hopkins R, Peden C, Gandhi S. *Radiology for anaesthesia and intensive care*. Cambridge University Press. 2002; 257–63.

## Question 6

a) What risk factors put a patient at risk of developing methicillin-resistant *Staphylococcus aureus* (MRSA) infection during a stay in hospital? (30%)
b) What preventive measures have been shown to be effective in minimising the spread of MRSA within a hospital? (60%)

### Additional Notes

MRSA is a huge problem in the NHS in terms of both the effect on patients and the high profile of 'superbug' stories in the media. It is, therefore, always a potential hot topic for examinations.

### Answer

a) Although there is now a significant proportion of people colonised with MRSA in the community (3%),✲ those at risk of developing morbidity and mortality from MRSA infections are still the group coming into hospital for invasive procedures.✲✲ As with most infections, the frail,✲ malnourished,✲ immuno-suppressed✲ and those at the extremes of age✲ are at a higher risk of developing clinical problems relating to MRSA. Patients are particularly at risk of MRSA if they:

 Have had previous colonisation with MRSA.✲
 Are admitted to an ICU.✲ Risk is proportional to length of stay.
 Have a higher APACHE II score.✲ This is proportional up to a score of 21, and then levels off.
 Have an intravascular device.✲ (9-fold increase)
 Are started on antibiotics,✲ with the risk increasing with number of antibiotics and duration of treatment.

b) The spread of MRSA may be prevented by:
 Reducing admission to hospital✲ and length of in-patient stay in hospital.✲
 Favouring non-invasive treatment modalities.✲
 Cleaning the environment.✲✲
  There are lots of studies showing correlations.
  MRSA is resistant to desiccation.
  May survive for 90 days on polyethylene.
  Dust control is important.

Handwashing.✷✷
 Alcohol rub at each bedside.✷
 Carried out between each patient.✷✷
 Should be performed effectively.✷ Compliance and technique are often poor.
Using either single-use or easy-to-decontaminate equipment.✷
Wearing disposable gloves during invasive procedures,✷✷ especially when examining wounds.✷✷ These should be thrown away with the dressing pack and the hands washed again. Dressings are not put onto patients' wounds while they are being washed or when the beds are being changed.✷
Disposable silicon covers on stethoscopes were introduced in Northern Ireland with some success.
Early screening of elective patients.✷✷ Patients testing positive should be treated with skin cleansers and oral antibiotics.✷ Basic infection-control measures should be used and, where resources allow, the patient should be isolated from other patients.✷
Screening staff. This is usually not recommended as it has questionable efficacy, with frequent recolonisation.
Using a separate ward for emergency patients.✷
Surgical antibiotic prophylaxis should be guided by protocol.✷ Antibiotics should only be given when absolutely necessary.✷✷ All patients testing positive or without a negative screening test result who require prophylactic antibiotics should be given a course that is sensitive against MRSA✷ (e.g. 3mg/kg gentamicin and 800mg teicoplanin). Screened negative patients requiring prophylaxis do not specifically need cover against MRSA.
Encouraging patients to complete courses of antibiotics.✷

### Reference
Hardy KJ, Hawkey PM, Gao F, Oppenheim BA. MRSA in the critically ill. *BJA* 2004; **92(1)**: 121–30.

## Question 7

a) What is the role of the National Institute for Clinical Excellence (NICE) and how does it develop a clinical guideline? (50%)
b) Name a recent NICE report that is of direct clinical relevance to anaesthetists or critical care doctors and outline the main findings. (40%)

### Additional Notes
There are a number of national organisations/reports that you need to know about for the exam. NICE, Confidential Enquiry into Maternal and Child Health (CEMACH), National Confidential Enquiry into Patient Outcome and Death (NCEPOD), National Patient Safety Agency (NPSA), recent AAGBI and Department of Health publications are all fair game for SAQ questions. Cochrane reviews are also extremely useful (type anaesthesia into the search engine at www.cochrane.org and you get over 600 hits!). There is considerable debate about whether NICE should be publishing best practice that is cost-independent and whether affordability should be decided by government.

### Answer
NICE is an independent✷ organisation responsible for providing national guidance✷ on promoting good health✷ and preventing and treating ill health.✷ It provides guidance in three main areas, public health, health technologies✷ and clinical practice✷; the latter two being of most relevance to anaesthetists.
NICE develops a guideline using the following steps:
A guideline topic is chosen✷✷
 Topic suggestions come from a variety of sources, e.g. clinicians,✷ the general public,✷ Department of Health.

Stakeholders register an interest✱
> e.g. patient groups, drug manufacturers, healthcare providers, statutory organisations.

Scope prepared✱
> i.e. what the guideline will or won't cover.

Guideline development group is established
> National Collaborating Centres (NCCs) established by NICE form these groups.

Draft guideline produced
Consultation on draft guideline
Final guideline produced and issued✱

b) There are a number of recent completed NICE reports. Awaited is their report into ultrasound-guided regional nerve block, due within the next year. An example of a recent report is:
*Technical patient safety solutions for ventilator associated pneumonia (VAP) in adults* (August 2008).
The two, key positive recommendations were:
> Mechanically ventilated, intubated patients should be nursed with their upper body elevated for as much time as possible.✱✱
> Oral antiseptics (e.g. chlorhexidine) should be included as part of the oral hygiene regime for all intubated, ventilated patients.✱✱ (You should know the key recommendations of the report you cite.)

Selective decontamination of the digestive tract (SDD) with topical antibiotics may reduce the incidence of VAP.✱ SDD with systemic antibiotics may also reduce mortality.✱ However, concerns were raised about causing an increase in *Clostridium difficile*✱ and selecting multi-resistant organisms.✱ The report suggested, therefore, more research into SDD.✱

There was inadequate robust evidence to make a recommendation on kinetic bed usage✱ or care bundles.✱

The report acknowledged that this is a difficult area of study as no definition✱ or diagnostic criteria✱ have been agreed upon for this condition. The overall scientific body of work in this field was poor, but the key recommendations were thought to be low risk for harm, backed up by evidence of efficacy and expert opinion.✱

### References

(All accessed on 30 December 2008.)
www.nice.org.uk
www.cochrane.org
www.aagbi.org
www.cemach.org.uk
www.ncepod.org.uk
Technical patient safety solutions for ventilator associated pneumonia in adults. Online at http://www.nice.org.uk/nicemedia/pdf/PSG002GuidanceWord.doc

## Question 8

a) Briefly describe the World Health Organization's (WHO) pain-relief ladder. (30%)
b) What cautions and contraindications are there to the prescription of non-steroidal anti-inflammatory drugs (NSAIDs)? (20%)
c) What advantages does a 1g dose of intravenous paracetamol have over a 1g oral dose of paracetamol when administered to an adult patient after general anaesthesia for four third molar extractions? (40%)

## Additional Notes
The first two sections of this question are core knowledge for anaesthetists and the marking scheme would have a relatively high proportion of essential information.

## Answer
a) The WHO pain-relief ladder describes an escalation of analgesia from simple analgesics for mild pain, adding in weak opiates for moderate pain and substituting them for stronger opiates for severe pain.★★
Drugs should be administered by the clock rather than on demand to maintain a pain-free state.★
See Figure 15 for the WHO pain-relief ladder:

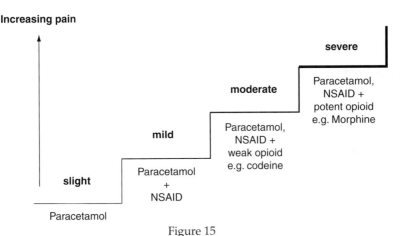

Figure 15

★★ for indicating escalating scale of pain
★★ for indicating an additive tactic where an additional agent is added on for the first three steps up the ladder
★★ each for indicating steps as being paracetamol, followed by NSAID, then weak opiate then substituted for strong opiate

b) Cautions for NSAID use are:
   Elderly★★
   Diabetic★
   Vascular disease★
   NSAID-sensitive asthma★★
   Renal failure★★
   Reduced urine output★
   Hypotension★
   Hypovolaemia★

   Contraindications to NSAID use are:
   Previous adverse/allergic reaction to NSAIDs★★
   History of peptic ulcer★★
   Already on another NSAID
   Oral anticoagulant therapy★
   Abnormal clotting★
   Current VTE prophylaxis with LMW heparin★

c) In some studies an IV dose of propacetamol equivalent to 1g of IV paracetamol was equianalgesic to 10mg morphine with fewer side effects.★

In a different study, enteral paracetamol had a Numbers Needed to Treat for molar extractions of 3.8.✷

Intravenous paracetamol provides:
    Ease of administration compared to swallowing tablets post extractions✷
    Earlier administration possible✷
    Guaranteed dose delivery regardless of emesis✷
    Faster onset of action from the point of administration✷✷
    Increased efficacy✷ (concentration effect at the blood/brain barrier)✷
    Increased bioavailability✷✷
    Reduced toxicity and side effects✷
    <100% of dose passed through the liver
    Guaranteed plasma level and dose closer to the toxic threshold, which is highly variable for paracetamol. With oral ingestion, toxicity seen in chronic use in some patients at 4g/day and fatality at 6g/day.

### References
Power I. Recent advances in postoperative pain therapy. *BJA* 2005; **95(1)**: 43–51.
WHO analgesia ladder. Online at http://www.who.int/cancer/palliative/painladder/en/ (Accessed 30 December 2008.)

## Question 9

a) What advice would you give a 35-year-old patient who is 8 weeks pregnant with acute appendicitis requiring surgery, when she asks you 'Will the anaesthetic affect my baby?' (40%)
b) A patient is 32 weeks into an uncomplicated pregnancy and develops acute, severe, neurological signs and symptoms requiring an urgent lumbar microdiscectomy. What are the specific problems in this case in relation to the pregnancy? (50%)

### Additional Notes
Part (a) is a common problem, the answer to which you should be familiar with. Part (b) requires you to use the knowledge that you have and apply it in a different setting. The examiners do not expect you to have experience of this case; they want to see that you can apply what you know.

### Answer
a) I would explain:
– Many of the drugs will cross your placenta and get to your baby.✷
– When babies need anaesthetics we give them the same drugs that we give to you.
– There is no evidence that the drugs affect the development of your baby or the chance of it developing a congenital abnormality.✷✷
– If you have a problem during the anaesthetic, e.g. low oxygen levels, then the baby can be harmed. For these reasons you will receive a style of anaesthetic which minimises this risk (antacid prophylaxis and RSI).✷✷
– Unrelated to the anaesthetic is the possibility that the operation or the appendicitis itself may increase the risk of abortion, growth restriction and low birth weight. The chance of this occurring reduces if we operate early.✷✷
– We will monitor the baby before and after surgery.

b) Two approaches:
1. GA for spinal surgery in the left lateral or prone positions with fetal monitoring.
2. LSCS preceding spinal surgery.
        Early discussion with anaesthetists, surgeons, obstetricians, midwives and neonatologists will define the approach.✷✷

Informed maternal consent is paramount in balancing the risks of fetal maturity vs maternal neurological outcome.★★

Problems:

Anaesthesia at 32/40

GA potentially hazardous (hypoxaemia, Mendelson's Syndrome)★

Fetal wellbeing

Morbidity from delivery at 32/40 gestation approximates 10%; mortality <5%
There is a 23% decrease in adverse outcome for each week that gestation continues between 32 and 39 weeks.
Can LSCS be delayed for 24 hours for the beneficial effects of steroids on fetal lung maturity?★
If LSCS does not precede neurosurgery, how will the fetus be monitored intraoperatively and what will be done about apparent fetal distress during a neurosurgical procedure?★★ Would tocolytics be required?
Are there SCBU beds or is transfer to another unit necessary?★

Maternal wellbeing

Patient positioning difficult given gravid uterus★★
Heightened risk of visceral ischaemia as uterine hypertrophy impairs visceral venous return★
Risk of placental hypoperfusion★★
Pressure areas at high risk★★
High risk of thrombosis★★ – needs anticoagulation but beware spinal haematoma

Surgery specific

X-rays/CT/MRI and dose exposure to the fetus★★
Possible large blood loss★
Raised venous pressure in Batsons plexus whilst prone increases bleeding into the surgical field★★

### References

Walton NKD, Melachuri VK. Anaesthesia for non-obstetric surgery during pregnancy. *Contin Educ Anaesth Crit Care Pain* 2006; **6**: 83–5.
Bastek JA, Sammel MD, Paré E, et al. Adverse neonatal outcomes: examining the risks between preterm, late preterm, and term infants. *Am J Obstet Gynecol* 2008; **199**: 367. e1–8.

## Question 10

a) List the causes of reduced conscious level in a 40-year-old male presenting to the Emergency Department. (30%)
b) What do you understand by the terms primary brain injury (PBI) and secondary brain injury (SBI) as applied to traumatic brain injury (TBI)?
   Outline pathophysiological mechanisms for both. (60%)

## Additional Notes

We wondered whether the final part of this question might be a bit tough until we discovered that primary and secondary brain injury is part of the syllabus for the surgical MRCS exam! The first part should be straightforward but does test your 'classify or die' technique to deliver a decent answer.

## Answer

a) Causes of reduced conscious level in this patient:

Primary brain problem

    Intracerebral bleed ✷

    Extradural haematoma ✷

    Subdural haematoma ✷

    Ischaemic stroke ✷

    Tumour ✷

    Head injury ✷✷

    Brain infection, e.g. meningitis or encephalitis ✷✷

Problems causing secondary brain dysfunction

Metabolic

    Hypo- or hyperglycaemia ✷✷

    Hepatic failure ✷✷

    Renal failure ✷

    Other electrolyte disturbances, e.g. hyponatraemia, hypocalcaemia ✷

    Hypothyroidism ✷

Infectious

    Systemic sepsis ✷✷

Drugs and poisons

    Alcohol ✷✷

    Sedatives ✷✷

    Illicit drugs ✷✷

Global physiological derangement

    Hypoxia ✷

    Hypercapnia ✷

    Status epilepticus ✷

    Post-ictal ✷

    Hypothermia/hyperthermia ✷

b) Primary brain injury:

Defined as the damage that occurs at the moment of trauma due to trauma associated with contact or the sequelae of the resulting acceleration–deceleration forces. ✷✷

This injury cannot be influenced by subsequent treatment. ✷

Can be focal or diffuse. ✷

Three main pathophysiological mechanisms of tissue damage due to:

    Tissue compression ✷

    Tissue stretching (tensile) ✷

    Tissue shearing ✷

Secondary brain injury (SBI):

Defined as injury that may develop over a period of hours or days following the initial traumatic injury. ✷✷ Some SBI may be inevitable while some may be preventable through avoidance of treatable causes, ✷ e.g. hypoxia, hypotension and hypercapnia.

SBI is a multi-factorial process mediated via a number of neurochemical mechanisms. ✷

Prevention of secondary injury is at the cornerstone of the intensive care management of the head-injured patient.

The main mediator of SBI is probably high intracellular calcium levels ✷ caused by a number of pathophysiological mechanisms including:

    Increase in circulating cytokines so enhancing the inflammatory response. ✷

    White matter damage. The part of the brain that provides axonal connections between different areas of grey matter is particularly sensitive to SBI.

Abnormal calcium homeostasis is central to this and to the ongoing damage seen in grey matter as well. Elevated intracellular calcium levels cause mitochondrial damage that ultimately leads to cell death.∗

Traumatic microvascular stenosis causes blood–brain barrier breakdown which causes cell swelling, membrane disruption and ultimately cell death.∗

Elevated levels of excitatory amino acids, e.g. aspartate and glutamate, are present after TBI and can directly cause cell death.∗

Increased AMPA-receptor and NMDA-receptor activation is seen in TBI and again mediates damage, predominantly via increased intracellular calcium concentration.∗

## References

Guidelines for the management of severe traumatic brain injury. *J Neurotrauma* 2007; **24** **(Supp I)**: S1–106

Park E, Bell J, Baker A. Traumatic brain injury: can the consequences be stopped? *CMAJ* 2008 April 22; **178(9):** 1163–70.

## Question 11

a) Regarding spinal anaesthesia what factors affect the spread of injected local anaesthetic solution? (70%)
b) What symptoms and signs would you expect to see in a patient with a high spinal blockade? (20%)

### Additional Notes

It is important to classify and classify some more with the first part of this question as there may be over 20 factors that can affect how high a spinal goes. There is some disagreement in the literature over some of the factors. It is probably worth stating this in your answer for extra brownie points. The second part is straightforward.

### Answer

a) Factors affecting spread of spinal anaesthesia can be divided into three main groups:

Characteristics of the injected solution∗∗
Operator technique∗∗
Patient characteristics∗∗

Characteristics of the injected solution:

Baricity (i.e. 'plain' or 'heavy' local anaesthetic solution).∗∗ Hyperbaric solutions are generally more predictable, with greater spread in the direction of gravity.∗

Volume∗∗ and dose.∗ There is not a linear relationship between dose increase and height of block (either for volume or concentration changes). However, within the range of doses normally used, a 50% increase in the injected dose will result in an increase in spread of approximately one dermatome. If the volume is kept constant and the 'dose' increased then there is a marginal increase in spread.

Operator technique:

Rapid injection of solution produces significantly greater spread of injection than a slower rate particularly for plain solutions.∗ The evidence for barbotage (repeated injection and aspiration of fluid) is equivocal.

Position of patient.∗∗ This has the greatest effect on spread of solution.

Needle position. There is conflicting evidence here. It may be that cephalad orientation of a Whitacre needle produces greater spread for a given dose of plain solution but not of a hyperbaric one.

Patient characteristics:

Height.✶ The taller the person the lower is the dermatome level reached for a given dose. Vertebral column length rather than height may be a more important determinant.

Cerebrospinal fluid (CSF) volume.✶ In patients with a decreased CSF volume, e.g. obstetric patients, the spread of solution is greater. Other CSF parameters, e.g. protein content, pressure and pH, have no effect.

Age.✶ In the very young and old there are small increases in spread of injected solution.

Weight. There is an argument that the obese have lower CSF volumes due to compression of the dural sac by epidural fat, so one would expect greater block height for a given dose. The evidence, particularly for plain solutions, is equivocal. Abnormal spinal anatomy may have a significant effect on spread.✶

b) A block extending above T4 is considered a high spinal.✶✶ The symptoms of a high spinal depend on the height of the block.✶

T1–T4 Bradycardia✶✶ due to block of sympathetic cardiac nerves✶ and worsening hypotension✶✶ due to peripheral vasodilatation secondary to complete (T1–L2) sympathetic nervous system blockade✶
C6–C8 Hand parasthesia and weakness✶✶
C3–C5 Diaphragmatic paralysis✶✶

Intracranial spread can also occur, leading to loss of consciousness✶✶ via a direct effect on the brain tissue.✶ This may also occur secondary to the hypotension (or apnoea!)

### References

Stienstra R, Veering B. Intrathecal drug spread: is it controllable? *Reg Anaesth Pain Med* 1998; **23**: 347–51.

Hocking G. Spinal anaesthetic spread. 2006. Online at http://www.frca.co.uk/article.aspx?articleid=100732. (Accessed on 3 January 2009.)

## Question 12

a) What criteria would lead you to consider starting renal replacement on a patient on the intensive care unit? (20%)
b) Describe the principles behind the filtration mechanism of the continuous renal replacement device used in your intensive care unit. (40%)
c) What are the risks of continuous renal replacement on the intensive care unit? (30%)

### Additional Notes

This question tests your understanding of renal replacement on the ICU. Much of the question can be answered through common sense and basic medical knowledge. However, the first question could be answered by a good medical student, so a poorly constructed answer here will do you no favours – construct your answer carefully.

You should understand the principles of osmosis and bulk flow as part of a renal replacement system and be able to describe the principles of continuous venovenous haemofiltration and haemodiafiltration, which are the common modalities used in the UK. A diagram here is useful; label it fully and provide a title – all of the labels given below would be regarded as essential. (✶✶ )

### Answer

a) Criteria may be:

Absolute:

Refractory pulmonary oedema✶✶

K$^+$ >6.9mmol/L★★
Metabolic acidosis pH<7.1★★
Uraemic symptoms (e.g. pericarditis – risks tamponade)★★
Relative:
Urea >35mmol/L★★
Creatinine >600mmol/L★★
Oliguria <5ml/kg per day★
Severe drug overdose known to be removed by filtration, e.g. salicylates★★
Hyperpyrexia★

b) See Figure 16.

### Continuous Venovenous Haemodiafiltration

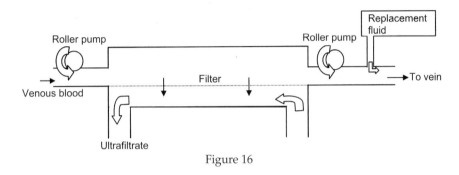

Figure 16

Blood is taken from and returned to a large vein by roller pumps (commonly 35 ml/kg per hr).★★
It passes along a semi-permeable membrane (the filter) which has a large surface area (>70m$^2$)★★ with pore size allowing passage of molecules of up to 30 000 Daltons.★
It is composed of polyacrylonitrile or polymethylmethacrylate.
Movement across the membrane is governed on the whole by Starling's law★★ :
$$\dot{Q} = k(P_b - P_u) - \sigma(\pi_b - \pi_u)$$★
($P$ = hydrostatic pressure, $\pi$ = colloid oncotic pressure, b = on blood side of membrane, u = on ultrafiltrate side of membrane, $k$ = filtration coefficient, $\sigma$ = reflection coefficient).

Movement of water and solutes is by three basic methods:
1. Ultrafiltration
   A hydrostatic driving force is set up across the membrane. This overcomes oncotic pressure, resulting in filtration of water and some solutes.★★
2. Diffusion
   Solutes and ions with molecular sizes smaller than filter pore size cross the membrane from high to low concentration (bidirectional); those with small molecular weights move more readily.★★
3. Convective transport
   The bulk movement of water molecules drags with it permeable, mid-sized solutes ('solute drag').★★

The countercurrent flow of ultrafiltrate ensures the gradient with the blood is maintained and more efficient filtration therefore results.★★

c) The risks can be subdivided into:
Those necessary for IV access:

Immediate

Arterial puncture, blood loss, haematoma★★

Puncture or damage of perivascular structures dependent on site:

    Nerve damage★★

    Lymphatic vessels

    Pneumothorax★★

    Tracheal/thyroid/bowel injury★★

    Wire-induced cardiac dysrrhythmias★

Early

    Line-related sepsis★★

    Thrombus/embolus★

Late

    Vessel stenosis (especially subclavian)★

Those relating to filtration:

    Blood loss (covert – in clotted filters, or overt if haemorrhage from port, e.g. from disconnection)★★

    Haemolysis★

    Risks of anticoagulation (e.g. GI haemorrhage or CVA) and heparin-induced thrombocytopenia★★

    Hypothermia, which may mask early signs of sepsis★

    Air embolus★

    Fluid depletion or overload★★

Other

    Drug clearance – may require dose adjustment

    Disequilibrium syndrome and cerebral oedema (more commonly seen with intermittent filtration)

## References

Deakin CD. Intensive care. In: *Clinical notes for the FRCA*, 2nd edition. Churchill Livingstone. 2000; 231–8.

Forni LG, Hilton PJ. Continuous hemofiltration in the treatment of acute renal failure. *N Engl J Med* 1997; **336**: 1303–9.

# Paper 8

Below are the model answers for this paper. ★★ indicates essential information, ★ indicates desirable information and unstarred text is supplementary information. As a guide, an answer with all the essential information and some desirable information would score 50% of the available points.

## Question 1

a) Draw a diagram showing the anatomy and relationships of the epidural space at the level of the tenth and eleventh thoracic vertebrae in the transverse plane. (40%)

b) Describe how you would seek consent for thoracic epidural analgesia in a patient listed for anterior resection. (50%)

**Additional Notes**

This is a potentially hazardous question. It would be very easy to run over the 15 minutes. Get the drawing and labels down in 6 minutes, then move on to the consent part. Put headings for the setting, the benefits, the risks, the alternatives and the question sections down and write lists or shortened notes under each heading.

**Answer**

a) A diagram showing the anatomy and relationships of the epidural space at the level of the tenth and eleventh thoracic vertebrae in the transverse plane
   See Figure 17.

b) The setting
   Ensure patient has capacity to understand. ★★
   Discuss preoperatively in clinic or on ward, ★ with patient un-premedicated. ★
   Procedure should be explained in lay terms appropriate to level of understanding of the patient. ★
   Printed material explaining the treatment and options in the patient's native language should be provided in advance of your conversation. ★

   The benefits
   Pain relief ★★ allowing the patient to deep breathe and cough, reducing risk of postoperative breathing problems. ★★
   Possible reduction in overall risk of death from operation but evidence is equivocal.
   Probably reduces risk of developing deep vein thrombosis. ★

   The risks
   Serious or frequently occurring risks should be explained. ★★

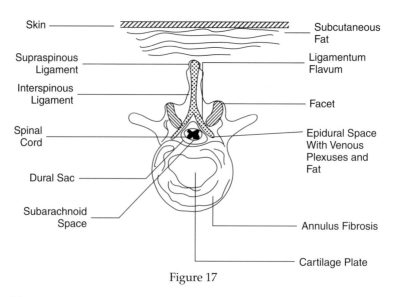

Skin — Subcutaneous Fat

Supraspinous Ligament — Ligamentum Flavum

Interspinous Ligament — Facet

Spinal Cord — Epidural Space With Venous Plexuses and Fat

Dural Sac

Subarachnoid Space — Annulus Fibrosis

Cartilage Plate

Figure 17

In this case:

Epidural may fail to provide complete pain relief.★

Epidurals commonly cause a reduction in blood pressure★★ which may reduce the blood supply to the healing gut and may require admission to high dependency for insertion of invasive monitoring and an infusion of drugs to raise the blood pressure.

Approximately 1 in 100 patients develop a headache.★★

The risk of temporary damage to a nerve is somewhere between 1 in 174 and 1 in 5000.★★

Permanent nerve damage occurs in somewhere between 1 in 5000 and 1 in 10 000 epidurals.★★

There is a risk of causing bleeding into★ or introducing infection★ into the epidural space. Whilst this is rare (quoted range from 1 in 1000 to 1 in 100 000) the consequences can be severe disability; in the worst cases paralysis can result.★★

Other options should be made clear to patient.★★

In this case:

The use of intravenous morphine usually via a patient-controlled device with the addition of regular simple pain-killers such as paracetamol and local anaesthetic into the wounds or around the nerves detecting pain such as a transversus abdominis plane block.★★

While studies suggest that overall pain control with a good epidural is better, in reality the difference is not that great and epidurals do not seem to reliably reduce any significant postoperative complications other than respiratory problems.★

The patient should then be given an opportunity to ask questions.★★

## References

AAGBI Guideline. Consent for anaesthesia, 2nd edition. 2006. Online at http://www.aagbi.org/publications/guidelines/docs/consent06.pdf (Accessed 1 January 2009.)

Grewal S, Hocking G, Wildsmith J. Epidural abscesses. *BJA* 2006; **96**(3): 292–302.

Low J, Johnston N, Morris C. Epidural analgesia: first do no harm. *Anaesthesia* 2008; **63**:1–3.

## Question 2

Outline the options for postoperative analgesia in a 71-year-old man who is undergoing pneumonectomy for adenocarcinoma of the lung. He has no other significant co-morbidities. (90%)

## Additional Notes

Many candidates will have had little exposure to thoracic anaesthesia prior to the final FRCA. However, questions do come up fairly frequently so it is important to have a good understanding of a number of issues in thoracic anaesthesia, especially one-lung ventilation. Remember analgesia post thoracotomy is not just a straight paravertebral catheter versus thoracic epidural answer. Think broad!

## Answer

Postoperative analgesia may never be more vital than after thoracic surgery. Ineffective analgesia may lead to significant morbidity in the short-term postoperative period ★★ and may also contribute towards chronic pain conditions ★ such as post-thoracotomy pain syndrome. Early, good, pain control may also avoid the 'wind up' phenomenon seen due to prolonged stimulation of the C fibres in the spinal cord dorsal horn. ★

Options for pain management, which should be used in combination, include:

  Systemic analgesics
  Neuroaxial techniques
  Regional anaesthetic techniques
  Other treatments

Systemic analgesics ★★

  The World Health Organisation (WHO) ladder for analgesia is a good basis for analgesic prescription. ★★
  Paracetamol should be given intravenously to ensure maximum bioavailability. ★
  NSAID use is warranted unless specifically contraindicated. ★
  Use of opiates depends on other techniques used in combination but if administered, a patient-controlled analgesia (PCA) machine is probably of benefit provided there has been adequate loading in the operative and immediate postoperative periods. ★
  Other analgesics to consider are clonidine (can be given either intravenously or epidurally), gabapentin (good evidence for an opioid sparing effect) and magnesium (equivocal evidence thus far but has potential).

Neuroaxial techniques ★★

  Both epidural and intrathecal routes can be used (individually or in combination as well in a combined spinal epidural technique). ★
  Opiates and local anaesthetic (LA) agents can be used alone or in combination. ★
  Probably provides better analgesia than systemic opiates alone, ★ provided the epidural is correctly sited ★ and is well managed. ★ These techniques may work well in combination with a systemic opiate PCA device.

Regional anaesthetic techniques

  There are a number of different techniques including:
    Intercostal nerve blocks ★★
    Single-shot technique that can be repeated ★
    Catheter insertion and LA infusion ★
    Intraoperative cryoablation of intercostal nerves
    Paravertebral nerve blocks ★★
    Either by multiple injections or catheter insertion and LA infusion ★

Other treatments

  A number of techniques may provide benefit, though in most cases scientific evidence is lacking. These include:
    Transcutaneous electrical nerve stimulation (TENS)
    Heat and cold application

Relaxation techniques
Hypnotherapy
Acupuncture

## References

Peeters-Asdourian C, Gupta S. Choices in pain management following thoracotomy. *Chest* 1999; **115**: 122–4. Online at http://www.chestjournal.org/cgi/reprint/115/suppl_2/122S (Accessed 1 January 2009.)
Vaughan R. Pain relief after thoracotomy. *BJA* 2001; **87**(5): 681–3. Online at http://bja.oxfordjournals.org/cgi/content/full/87/5/681 (Accessed 1 January 2009.)

## Question 3

a) Outline the clotting cascade and use it to illustrate the mechanism of action of recombinant factor VIIa. (40%)
b) When might recombinant factor VIIa prove of benefit in clinical practice? (15%)
c) Explain what happens to this cascade in the development of disseminated intravascular coagulopathy (DIC). (35%)

### Additional Notes

There has been lots of hype about recombinant factor VIIa. You will find yourself in situations where its use is considered, therefore you should know how it works.

The College has, in a similar fashion, asked a question on Sugammadex in 2008, so a question such as this is not beyond the bounds of possibility.

### Answer

a) Clotting cascade

Figure 18 shows the revised view of the coagulation cascade. It has gained popularity as it overcomes some of the paradoxes of the classic coagulation cascade.

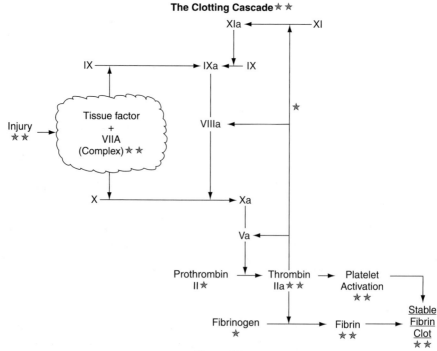

**The Clotting Cascade** ★ ★

Figure 18

The initiating event in haemostasis is the exposure of tissue factor (TF) and formation of the TF/VIIa complex.★★
Recombinant factor VIIa (rFVIIa) enhances the TF pathway, directly activating factor X to Xa. In the presence of factor Va, this leads to an increase in thrombin generation which in turn activates platelets.★★
The activated platelets, in the presence of factors VIIIa and Va, now generate large volumes of thrombin, amplifying its production – the 'thrombin burst'.★
Increased levels of thrombin have a positive effect on factors higher up the clotting cascade, which propagates clot production.★★

b) Clinical use

rFVIIa is licensed for bleeding in patients with:
    Haemophilia with antibodies to factors VIII and IX★★★
    Factor VII deficiency★★★
    Glanzmann thrombasthenia refractory to platelet transfusion★★

'Off-licence' use of rFVIIa has been the source of much research and controversy over recent years.
A recent Cochrane review suggests some possible benefit of rFVIIa in intracranial haemorrhage but the evidence for all other off-licence indications is extremely weak.★
There is no evidence to recommend its prophylactic use in surgery.★
If used, it should be reserved for microvascular ooze in patients with normal pH, temperature and fibrinogen, whose platelets are $>50\times10^{9}$/L.★

c) DIC
The pathological activation of the coagulation cascade leading to a consumptive coagulopathy and fibrinolysis, usually secondary to one of several causes, e.g. shock, sepsis, placental abruption.★
Platelets and clotting factors are consumed by the pathological process during the formation of microthrombi.★★
This activates the fibrinolytic system, which generates plasmin.
Plasmin breaks down fibrinogen and fibrin and inhibits the action of factors V and VIII, reducing the thrombin-forming capabilities of the cascade.★★
Fibrin degradation products are produced which are themselves inhibitory to the coagulation cascade and to platelets.★
A dwindling number of platelets and clotting factors therefore have their action inhibited by overactivation of the fibrinolytic system.★★

## References

Roberts HR, Monroe DM, Miguel A, et al. Current concepts of haemostasis. Implications for therapy. *Anesthesiology* 2004; **100**: 722–30.
Ridley S, Taylor B, Gunning K. Medical management of bleeding in critically ill patients. *Contin Educ Anaesth Crit Care Pain* 2007; **7**: 116–21.
Stanworth S, Birchall J, Doree C, et al. Recombinant factor VIIa for the prevention and treatment of bleeding in patients without haemophilia. *Cochrane review*. http://www.cochrane.org/reviews/en/ab005011.html. (Accessed 12 November 2008.)
Greaves M. Blood and bone marrow. In: Underwood JCE ed. *General and systematic pathology*, 2nd edition.Churchill Livingstone. 1996: 740–742.

## Question 4

a) What is the mechanism by which hypoxia can precipitate a sickle cell crisis? (30%)
b) What are the anaesthetic considerations in the perioperative period when anaesthetising a known HbSC patient undergoing elective knee replacement? (60%)

## Additional Notes

Sickle cell disease (SCD) is one of those things the College like to ask about because it is a disease which has multi-system implications.

Remember SCD refers to a group of haemoglobinopathies and not just the homozygote (HbSS) disease. Heterozygote HbS carriers (HbAS or sickle cell trait) can exist alone or with other β-chain abnormalities (compound heterozygous states) such as haemoglobin C (HbSC disease), haemoglobin D (HbSD disease) or β-thalassaemia (HbS/β-thal disease).

In terms of disease severity HbSC lies somewhere between HbSS and HbAS.

## Answer

a) Mechanism of hypoxia:

Deoxygenated HbS loses its ability to deform easily.✶✶ This leads to vascular obstruction✶✶ and as a result tissue ischaemia.✶✶

In addition there is considerable evidence that the vascular endothelium in these patients is abnormal✶ and that this abnormality makes the patient with SCD more vulnerable to hypoxia. This abnormality causes an imbalance in vasomotor tone✶ causing vasoconstriction,✶ increased circulating inflammatory molecules✶ (e.g. interleukin-1, C-reactive protein and tumour necrosis factor) and importantly thrombin production,✶ so worsening the tissue ischaemia.

These patients may also have impaired oxygen delivery✶ secondary to pulmonary damage✶ and raised blood viscosity.✶

b) Anaesthetic considerations:

Postoperative complication rates of up to 18% have been reported in this patient group, so meticulous care is required.✶

Preoperatively, close liaison with the haematology team is essential.✶ It is vital to send blood for crossmatch early as antibody production in this group is common.✶ The requirement for exchange transfusion depends on the individual patient and the surgery needed.✶

Patients with HbSC disease are prone to anaemia,✶ bone marrow and splenic infarcts✶ (40% of adults are asplenic), cerebrovascular disease,✶ hepatic disease✶ and renal impairment.✶ Hence a full set of bloods (FBC, U + E, LFTs, bone profile) is essential in all patients.✶✶

Potential problems are hypoxia,✶✶ dehydration,✶✶ infection✶ (especially Gram-negative bacteria✶), acidosis,✶ hypothermia✶✶ and pain.✶✶ These should be considered within an extended perioperative period. Postoperative high-dependency unit admission may be beneficial.✶

Intraoperative use of tourniquets is relatively contraindicated✶ though with meticulous limb exsanguination, maintenance of hydration and acid-base status successful tourniquet use has been described.

Prevention of hypothermia should begin preoperatively before the patient leaves the ward.✶ Theatre temperature should be monitored closely and the use of forced air and fluid warmers is essential.✶✶ A low threshold for an arterial line and intraoperative cardiac output monitoring (e.g. oesophageal Doppler) to monitor acid base, oxygenation and fluid status is important✶ as is antibiotic prophylaxis.✶ Regional blockade to reduce pain and also increase flow by sympathetic blockade should be considered.✶

Intraoperative sickle crises may be hard to detect.✶

Postoperative pain control may be difficult as these patients may already be opiate-tolerant.✶

## References

Firth P. Anaesthesia for peculiar cells – a century of sickle cell disease. *BJA* 2005 **95(3):** 287–299. Online at http://bja.oxfordjournals.org/cgi/reprint/aei129v1?ck=nck (Accessed 29 December 2008.)

Haxby E, Bateman C. Anaesthesia for patients with sickle cell disease. *Anaesth Intensive Care Med* 2004; **5(3):** 95–6.

## Question 5

a) What are the specific preoperative concerns one might have in a 35-year-old lady with known systemic lupus erythematosus (SLE) who is presenting for laparoscopic cholecystectomy? (60%)
b) List the potential complications of corticosteroid treatment commonly used in patients with this condition? (30%)

### Additional Notes
The College enjoys asking questions about patients presenting for anaesthesia who suffer from a disease with multi-system manifestations. It allows a good candidate to give a well-structured answer and opens up a number of question angles. SLE, commonest in young females, is characterised by autoantibody production which manifests in a number of ways secondary to immune-mediated tissue damage. Remember there is a drug-induced form of the disease.

### Answer
Preoperative concerns are related to the clinical manifestations of the disease and the problems associated with the drugs used in its treatment. The main anaesthetic implications are related to cardiovascular disease, renal disease and coagulation status.

Cardiovascular disease:✶✶
  Pericarditis can occur in 60%,✶ myocarditis in 15% of patients and non-bacterial endocarditis (so called Libman-Sachs endocarditis) affecting the mitral and aortic valves in up 25%.✶
  Raynaud's phenomenon is common and accelerated atherosclerotic disease occurs.✶
  Pleural effusions, interstitial fibrosis, pulmonary vasculitis, pulmonary embolism and interstitial pneumonitis occur in up to 20%.✶
  Hypertension may be present and is usually secondary to renal impairment.✶

Renal disease:✶✶
  Renal impairment is common secondary to glomerulonephritis and patients are commonly nephrotic.✶

Coagulation status:✶✶
  Anaemia of chronic disease, immune thrombocytopaenia and hypercoagulable states are the hallmarks of patients with SLE.✶
  Antiphospholipid antibody (also known as the lupus anticoagulant) occurs in up to a third of patients. This may prolong the APTT but paradoxically is associated with increased risk of recurrent arterial and venous thrombotic events.✶
  Other antibodies to coagulation proteins, e.g. factor VIII and prothrombin, predispose the patient to haemorrhage.

Other systems:
  More than 50% of SLE patients have some form of neuropsychiatric abnormality.✶
  Plasma cholinesterase activity may be impaired.✶
  Arthritis and arthralgia are common.

Drugs:✶✶
  There are a number of immunosuppressive strategies for the treatment of SLE. Drugs used include corticosteroids, cyclophosphamide, azathioprine, ciclosporin and methotrexate.
  Patients may undergo plasmapheresis.

b) Complications of steroid therapy include:

    Mineralocorticoid related✷✷ – hypokalaemia, fluid retention, hypertension
    Hyperglycaemia and diabetes mellitus✷✷
    Peptic ulcer disease✷
    Osteoporosis✷
    Cushing's syndrome✷
    Adrenal suppression✷
    Infection✷
    Decreased wound healing✷
    Myopathy
    Growth suppression in children
    Pancreatitis
    CNS symptoms, including depression, euphoria, psychosis and insomnia

### References

Rahman A, Isenberg D. Systemic lupus erythematosus. *NEJM* 2008; **358**: 929–39.
Davies S. Systemic lupus erythematosus and the obstetrical patient – implications for the anaesthetist. *Canad J Anaesth* 1991; **38**: 790–6. Online at http://www.cja-jca.org/cgi/reprint/38/6/790 (Accessed 31 December 2008.)

## Question 6

At pre-assessment clinic a patient for rhinoplasty informs you that he has smoked 20 cigarettes a day for the last 20 years. He is thinking about quitting smoking. He asks whether it is a good idea to stop before the surgery or to wait until the operation is out of the way. What advice would you give him? (90%)

### Additional Notes

Answering a 'patient advice' question is daunting to some candidates. Should your answer be a narrative of the discussion or reported speech? Should you write in lay terms? I think the style used here is preferable. It is unlikely that marks will be available for discussing the reduction in cytokine expression in smokers.

### Answer

The emphatic answer to the patient should be 'Yes, it would definitely be beneficial for you to stop smoking before your operation.✷✷ Stopping smoking has been shown to reduce the risk of postoperative complications,✷✷ especially if for at least 6 weeks before surgery.'✷

I would try to convey as much of the following to the patient as they would be able to assimilate in one meeting, using lay language✷ or explanations to aid understanding. ✷ This can be enhanced by encouraging someone to attend with the patient, asking the patient to tell you what they understand you have said to them and by handing them a relevant leaflet to take away.✷

If he stops smoking he is less likely to:

- have complications such as dehiscence of the surgical wound✷✷
- suffer breathing problems such as chest infection in the postoperative period✷✷
- have circulation and heart complications such as myocardial infarction postoperatively✷✷
- have complications related to the gastrointestinal and musculoskeletal systems along with more risk of infections.

Stopping 12 hours before surgery significantly reduces the level of carboxyhaemoglobin, increases oxygen-carrying capacity of your blood, and reduces the negative inotropic and arrhythmic effects of smoking.✷✷

Stopping 12–24 hours before will reduce increased heart rate and blood pressure and improve peripheral vasoconstriction.✷
A week will improve raised blood viscosity and polycythaemia.✷
One month improves small airway function, which continues to improve for a further 6 months.✷
Six weeks will produce gains in reducing excess sputum production, with 50% reduction in the first 2 weeks.✷✷
Two months reduces the risk of postoperative chest infection, with risk approaching that of non-smokers if he stops for 6 months.✷
The longer the period of abstinence, the less likely is a wound complication.✷

He should be advised about the importance of staying off smoking once the operation is over.✷✷ This will reduce his risk from postoperative complications such as myocardial infarction.
He should be advised that his GP will have access to a range of advice and resources that will help him stop smoking.✷ He should be encouraged that by actively wanting to stop smoking, he is in a group who are more likely to be successful at quitting cigarettes.

### References
BMA's tobacco control website at http://www.tobacco-control.org/ (Accessed 1 January 2009.)
Kuri M, Nakagawa M, Tanaka H, Hasuo S, Kishi Y. Determination of the duration of preoperative smoking cessation to improve wound healing after head and neck surgery. *Anesthesiology* 2005; **102**: 892–6.

## Question 7

a) Define sepsis. (15%)
b) In the Surviving Sepsis Campaign, what are the key points in the resuscitation bundle (25%) and in the management bundle? (20%)
c) What is the point of providing care bundles (15%) and how have they been criticised? (15%)

### Additional Notes
At the time of writing a question on sepsis had never been asked in the SAQs. Given that on ICU you will be expected to deal with septic patients on a daily basis, this is almost unbelievable. Know the basics and be prepared!

### Answer
a) Sepsis is defined as the systemic response to infection. It requires the presence of:

1. Infection (the inflammatory response to the presence of microorganisms or invasion of a normally sterile site by these organisms),✷✷ and
2. The systemic inflammatory response system, i.e. two or more of:
     Temperature >38°C or <36°C✷✷
     Heart rate >90/min✷✷
     Respiratory rate >20 or $PaCO_2$ <32mmHg✷✷
     White cells >12 000/mm³ or <400/mm³ or the presence of >10% immature forms✷✷

b) Resuscitation bundle
     Must occur within the first 6 hours of identification of severe sepsis✷
     Measure serum lactate✷✷
     Obtain blood cultures prior to antibiotic administration✷✷
     Administer broad-spectrum antibiotics within 3 hours of ED admission and within 1 hour of non-ED admission✷✷

If hypotension or serum lactate >4mmol/L
   Minimum 20ml/kg crystalloid bolus or equivalent★★
   If remains hypotensive, vasopressors so MAP >65mmHg★★
If hypotension persists despite fluid resuscitation (septic shock) or lactate >4mmol/L:
   Insert central line and aim for CVP >8mmHg★
   Aim for central venous $O_2$ sats >70% or mixed venous $O_2$ sats >65%★

Management bundle
Must begin immediately★
   Administer low-dose steroids 200–300mg/day if unresponsive to fluid and
   vasopressors★★
   Administer recombinant human activated protein C (rhAPC) if APACHE II >25
   and multi-organ failure★★
   Maintain glucose >4.2 and <8.3mmol/L★★
   If ventilated – peak inspiratory pressure <30cmH$_2$O★★

c) The aim of care bundles is to reduce ICU mortality.
They are a group of interventions that when implemented together result in better outcomes than when implemented individually.★★
They provide a 'package' of care, each aspect of which has been scrutinised by expert opinion.
These bundles:
   Minimise the chance that important aspects of sepsis care are neglected.★★
   Provide a structure of care, day or night to staff of varying grades.
   Encourage the practice of evidence-based medicine.★
   Where this is not available, expert opinion is exercised.
   Provide a benchmark of care and therefore a standard against which a unit may audit its practice.★

They have been criticised because:
   Manufacturers of activated protein C have been heavily involved in funding the campaign.★
   Evidence for universal use of rhAPC is dwindling.★★
   The evidence supporting the use of bundles is limited.

### References

Surviving sepsis campaign: www.survivingsepsis.org. (Accessed on 27 October 2008.)
Fletcher S. The Surviving Sepsis Campaign and sepsis care bundles: substance or sophistry. *Anaesthesia* 2006; **61**: 313–5.
Rivers E, Nguyen B, Havstad S, et al. Early goal-directed therapy in the treatment of severe sepsis and septic shock. *N Engl J Med* 2001; **345**: 1368–77.

## Question 8

With reference to medical statistics, define and illustrate with clinical examples the following terms:
a) Normal distribution. (20%)
b) Type I and type II error. (30%)
c) Sensitivity and specificity. (40%)

### Additional Notes

Most people shudder at the idea of ever being asked a statistics question. It does, however, form part of the syllabus for the FRCA so you would be unwise not to approach it in your revision at some point, albeit reasonably close to the exam (to avoid forgetting it). Six continuing-education journals from the RCOA in 2007–2008 contained topics on statistics, so it is clearly thought to be important. That alone should persuade you to ensure you know the basics well and be familiar with some relevant tests and statistical principles, as asked in this question.

## Answer

a) Normal distribution

Refers to quantitative data where the mean, median and mode are equal.★★
Also referred to as a Gaussian or parametric distribution.★
Yields a unimodal bell-shaped curve when frequency is plotted against interval data.★★ See Figure 19.

**Normal Distribution, Showing Standard Deviations (SD)** ★★

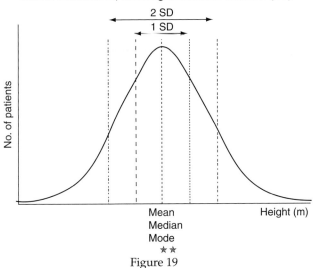

Figure 19

E.g. In the measurement of height of clinic patients:
68% of the patients lie within 1 standard deviation (1 SD) of the central tendency.★★
95% of patients lie within 2 standard deviations (2 SD) of the central tendency.★★
These are other features of normally distributed data.

b) Type I error

A statistically significant difference is found between two groups when none actually exists.★★
Statistical analysis has erroneously yielded a $p$ value of <0.05; the chance of this occurrence is 5% at this probability level.

Type II Error
No statistically significant difference between the groups is found where one does actually exist.★★
Statistical analysis has erroneously yielded a p value of >0.05.
The most common cause for a type II error is inadequate sample size.★★
To avoid this, a study should be adequately powered.★
The power of a study is $(1 - \beta) \times 100\%$, $\beta$ being the probability of a type II error.
A power of >80% is acceptable.

c) Sensitivity and specificity

These are measures of the performance of a diagnostic test.★★
Sensitivity represents the ability of a test to correctly report all positive findings.★★
Specificity represents the ability of a test to correctly report all negative findings.★★

These can be represented mathematically as below.

E.g. the fire alarm in my hospital goes off frequently. It always sounds when there is a fire, but often sounds when there is not a fire:

Table 4. *Sensitivity and specificity*

|  |  | Fire | |
| --- | --- | --- | --- |
|  |  | Present | Absent |
| Alarm | Rings | a | b |
|  | Silent | c | d |

Sensitivity = a/a+c✶
Specificity = d/d+b✶

In this example, this fire alarm is highly sensitive but poorly specific.

Screening tests must be highly sensitive to pick up patients with disease. Patients will then go on to have further tests so a screening specificity of <100% is acceptable. Sensitivity and specificity are independent of the population of interest (unlike positive and negative predictive values).✶

### References

Mccluskey A, Lalkhen AG. Statistics II. *Contin Educ Anaesth Crit Care Pain* 2007; **7**: 128–30.

McCluskey A, Lalkhen AG. Statistics IV.*Contin Educ Anaesth Crit Care Pain* 2007; **7**: 208–12.

Lalkhen AG, McCluskey A. Clinical tests: sensitivity and specificity. *Contin Educ Anaesth Crit Care Pain* 2008; **8**: 221–3.

## Question 9

a)  What is the definition of status epilepticus? (20%)
b)  List the possible causes. (30%)
c)  Outline your initial management of the convulsing patient presenting in the Emergency Department. (40%)

### Additional Notes

This has, perhaps surprisingly, not come up as a question in the SAQ part of the exam before. It is a big topic but one that can be classified easily. Remember presentation of status epilepticus (SE) is not exclusively grand mal and think about treating the patient not just the seizure as part of your answer.

### Answer

a) The World Health Organisation defines SE as 'A condition characterised by an epileptic seizure that is sufficiently prolonged✶✶ or repeated✶✶ at sufficiently brief intervals✶✶ so as to produce an unvarying and enduring✶✶ epileptic condition'. Some other definitions use a defined time span for the seizure,✶ e.g. greater than 5 minutes for a single seizure or group of seizures with no recovery in between.

It is important to note that a patient may be in SE but not be having grand mal seizure activity. SE can therefore be divided into generalised convulsive status epilepticus (GCSE) and non-convulsive status epilepticus (NCSE).

b)  Causes of SE can be divided into:
   Causes in patients with a history of epilepsy
      Traumatic brain injury✶✶
      Alcohol✶✶

Infection✳
Sub-therapeutic anticonvulsant levels✳

Causes in patients with no history of epilepsy
Cerebrovascular event✳✳ (infarct, haemorrhage including subarachnoid)
Hypoxic brain injury, e.g. post cardiac arrest✳
Intracranial space-occupying lesion✳
Traumatic brain injury✳✳
Drugs.✳✳ Overdose,✳ withdrawal✳✳ (especially alcohol) and illicit use,
    e.g. amphetamines
Electrolyte abnormalities✳ (hypo- and hypernatraemia, hypercalcaemia,
    hypoglycaemia)
Hepatic encephalopathy✳
Eclampsia✳✳
Infection✳✳
Vasculitis

c) Initial management centres on an Airway, Breathing, Circulation approach.✳✳

The plan is to maintain oxygenation,✳✳ terminate seizures✳✳ and identify and treat the underlying cause.✳✳ Airway control may be achieved by simple airway manoeuvres alone.✳
A brief history from a witness may be invaluable.✳
Attach patient to appropriate monitoring,✳ insert intravenous access✳ and send appropriate bloods, which will include all or some of the following: FBC, U+Es,✳ glucose,✳ toxicology screen,✳ anticonvulsant levels,✳ blood alcohol,✳ LFTs, calcium. Check temperature.✳

Seizure termination:
    Treatment of underlying cause✳✳ e.g. oxygen for hypoxia, glucose for hypogly-caemia, magnesium for eclampsia.

Drug therapies:
    Remember buccal and rectal routes if cannulation is impossible.✳
    Lorazepam✳✳ 4mg IV is longer-acting with better anticonvulsant activity than diazepam.
    Phenytoin✳✳ 15mg/kg loading dose at no more than 50mg/min.
    If the above fail then consider induction of anaesthesia and intubation.✳✳ This allows second-line treatment of SE, for example.

    Propofol (induction dose then 2–10mg/kg/hr maintenance)✳
    Thiopentone 1–5mg/kg/hr✳
    Phenobarbitone 5–12mg/kg✳

Gold standard would be for continual EEG monitoring while under anaesthesia.✳ CT scanning may be appropriate if diagnosis remains unclear✳ and should be done en route to critical care to minimise transfers.

### References
Walker M. Status epilepticus: an evidence based guide. *BMJ* 2005; **331**: 673–7. Online at http://www.bmj.com/cgi/content/full/331/7518/673 (Accessed 28 December 2008.)
Chapman M, Smith M, Hirsch N. Status epilepticus. *Anaesthesia* 2002; **56**(7): 648–59.

## Question 10

a) What is the difference between decontamination, cleaning, disinfection and steri-lisation? (30%)
b) List the techniques used for sterilisation of medical equipment. (30%)

c) Describe how a reusable Classic Laryngeal Mask Airway™(LMA) is decontaminated prior to it being safe to use again. (30%)

## Additional Notes

It was the prion scare that made the decontamination and reuse of equipment frontline news. No decontamination technique is 100% guaranteed to remove prions. The potential prion risk has decreased and as always there are cost pressures to consider when balancing single use with multi-use equipment. If the topical view swings back towards multi-use, then how items are cleaned becomes a hot topic.

## Answer

a) Decontamination

A combination of processes✶ which removes and/or destroys✶ contamination so that infectious agents or other contaminants cannot initiate infection✶ or other harmful response. It is carried out in the following ways:

Cleaning

The physical removal of foreign material.✶✶ Cleaning physically removes rather than kills microorganisms. Thorough and meticulous cleaning is required before any equipment can be disinfected or sterilised.✶

Disinfection

The inactivation of disease-producing microorganisms.✶✶ Disinfection does not destroy bacterial spores.✶

Sterilisation

This is the level of reprocessing required when processing medical equipment/devices.✶✶ Sterilisation results in the destruction of all forms of microbial life, including bacteria, spores, viruses and fungi.✶✶

b) Sterilisation can be carried out in a number of ways including:

Steam✶✶

This is often done under pressure in an autoclave✶ to reduce sterilisation time, e.g. 30min at 1 atmosphere 122°C or 10min at 1.5 atmospheres 126°C.

There are different methods of autoclave, e.g. prevacuum or gravity displacement.

Steam and formaldehyde ('low-temperature' steam method)✶

Hot air (i.e. 'dry heat')✶

6% hydrogen peroxide

2% glutaraldehyde✶

Ethylene oxide✶

Irradiation✶ (tends to be confined to large-scale commercial use)

c) Decontaminating an LMA is a step-by-step process.✶✶ Remember sterilisation cannot take place unless cleaning has taken place first.✶

Step 1.   Wash the LMA✶✶

This should be done in warm water with a mild detergent or a dilute sodium bicarbonate solution.✶ Use a soft bristle brush to clean any residue from the lumen of the tube.✶

It is important to avoid exposure of the LMA to a cleaning solution such as iodine, glutaraldehyde or anything phenol-based which may damage the LMA.✶

Step 2.   Rinse and dry the LMA✶

Step 3.   Inspect the LMA to ensure all visible foreign matter has been removed and repeat steps 1 and 2 if necessary✶

Step 4.   Steam autoclave the LMA✶✶

Step 5.   Record LMA sterilisation on card supplied with each reusable LMA✶

## References

Sterilisation and decontamination of medical devices. Online at http://www.mhra.gov.uk/safetyinformation/generalsafetyinformationandadvice/technicalinformation/sterilizationanddecontaminationofmedicaldevices/index.htm (Accessed 1 January 2009.)

National Resource for Infection Control (NRIC). Online at http://www.nric.org.uk. (Accessed 1 January 2009.)

## Question 11

a) List the contraindications to regional anaesthesia for phacoemulsification of cataract surgery. (40%)
b) What are the potential advantages of sub-Tenon's anaesthesia versus topical anaesthesia for cataract surgery? (50%)

### Additional Notes

Considering how many ophthalmic procedures anaesthetists are involved in it is perhaps surprising that the College has not focused (pardon the pun) more on SAQs with an ophthalmic anaesthesia slant. There are increasing numbers of cataracts being extracted under topical anaesthesia alone and there has been a recent Cochrane review. The examiners are always on the lookout for sources of new questions and the Cochrane database is one of their hunting grounds. Due to the risks of globe perforation, optic nerve damage and even brainstem anaesthesia 'sharp needle techniques' (i.e. peri- and retrobulbar blocks) are becoming less popular.

### Answer

a) There are few absolute contraindications to a regional technique for phaco surgery, with patient refusal despite counselling and an explanation of the risks involved being the only absolute.✶✶ For the following each patient needs to be assessed on an individual basis.

Relative contraindications:
   The confused patient who is unable to comply with instructions, unable to communicate or whose safety may be compromised.✶✶
   The patient with marked, uncontrolled tremor.✶
   A patient with a medical condition that prevents acceptable positioning.✶ (The thought of then offering that patient a general anaesthetic is often not appealing!)
   The young patient.✶ There is no absolute age below which local anaesthesia is contraindicated.
   A patient who has experienced an allergic reaction or complication to local anaesthetic in the past.

b) The advantages of topical anaesthesia are:
   Shorter administration time.✶✶
   Shorter duration of action (so allowing the patient to more rapidly regain sight after surgery).
   Less pain during administration.✶
   No chemosis.✶
   No conjunctival haemorrhage.

   Advantages of sub-Tenon's anaesthesia
   Better surgical conditions due to akinesia and reduction in lid movements.✶✶
   Some evidence of surgical preference for a sub-Tenon's technique possibly related to operating on a more akinetic eye.✶
   Better patient satisfaction.✶✶
   Lower pain scores.✶✶

Reduction in surgical complications.✶✶ Posterior capsule tear and vitreous loss occurred more than twice as often in the topical group in currently published data. Allows surgeon more scope to proceed if any complications were to occur during the procedure.✶

May allow better operating conditions for more junior surgeons.

### References

The Royal College of Anaesthetists and The Royal College of Ophthalmologists, Local Anaesthesia for Intraocular Surgery. 2001. Online at www.rcoa.ac.uk/docs/RCARCOGuidelines.pdf (Accessed 27 December 2008.)

Davison M, Padroni S, Bunce C, Rüschen H. Sub-Tenon's anaesthesia versus topical anaesthesia for cataract surgery. *Cochrane Database of Systematic Reviews* 2007, Issue 3. Art. No.: CD006291. Online at http://www.cochrane.org/reviews/en/ab006291.html (Accessed 3 January 2009.)

## Question 12

a) A woman in labour has an epidural in situ. Unfortunately she is experiencing moderate (6/10) pain with contractions. This is predominantly rightsided in a T10–T12 distribution. Outline your management. (50%)

b) Six hours later the same woman needs to go to theatre for a trial of instrumental delivery as the CTG shows late decelerations. She has received an infusion of local anaesthetic / fentanyl mix with no bolus doses within the last 2 hours. Her epidural is again patchy – what are your options? (40%)

### Additional Notes

Although this question is about a situation you will have been in many times working on the delivery suite, the answer needs to be thought about carefully. The temptation to waffle should be resisted, and think carefully about where the extra marks will be awarded.

### Answer

a) A missed segment during a contraction is often due to a unilateral block.

Firstly, perform an initial assessement. This will include:

A visual inspection of catheter site for catheter slippage/leakage.✶✶

An examination of the epidural administration chart for recent bolus dose administration and infusion rate.✶

Determining the stage of labour reached.✶✶

Checking the block height.✶✶

A discussion with the patient.✶✶This involves an assessment of how severe the pain is✶✶ and communicating the potential options to improve it.✶✶ This will depend on pain severity, patient choice, anticipated duration of labour and potential for caesarean section / instrumented delivery. The patient may be happy to continue as things are. Other analgesic options can be considered.✶✶

If the patient wants the epidural improved then a management plan could be:

Epidural top up✶ with patient right side (i.e. 'bad side') down.✶ Top-up can be a bolus of the epidural solution and can include additional opiate, e.g. fentanyl 50–100μg.✶

If that fails then withdrawing the catheter by 1–2cm and re-bolusing may help.✶✶

If that fails, the patient is still uncomfortable and they are aware of the risks associated with resiting the epidural (dural puncture etc.)✶ and there is no imminent need for a caesarean section / instrumental delivery✶ then the epidural should be resited.✶✶

b) This is a slightly different situation as the need for excellent analgesia (S5–T4) is paramount.✶✶ Again maternal involvement in the decision-making process is vital so a concise conversation covering all issues is essential. ✶✶ Speak to the obstetric team to get an indication of precise timescales regarding delivery. ✶ Repeat examination of catheter site, sensory level and epidural chart should be carried out if time permits. ✶ The potential options are:

Bolus dose of local anaesthetic +/− opiate solution e.g. 20ml total including 2% lidocaine, 1ml of 8.4% sodium bicarbonate and 1ml 1 in 10 000 epinephrine. Additional opiate, e.g. 50–100μg fentanyl, can also be added. There is an argument that one should never try to bolus a patchy epidural prior to delivery/ caesarean. ✶

Switch to spinal anaesthetic. ✶✶ Most people would reduce the dose of spinal anaesthetic if a bolus dose has been given down the epidural but it depends on degree of patchiness. ✶

Resite epidural. ✶

General anaesthetic. ✶ This is probably the least desirable option. ✶

## References

Allman K, Wilson I. Anaesthesia for caesarean section. *Oxford handbook of anaesthesia.* Oxford University Press. 2006; 711–21.

Urqhart J, Plaat F, Collis R. *Textbook of obstetric anaesthesia.* Greenwich Medical Media. 2002; 133–50.

# Paper 9

Below are the model answers for this paper. ★★ indicates essential information, ★ indicates desirable information and unstarred text is supplementary information. As a guide, an answer with all the essential information and some desirable information would score 50% of the available points.

## Question 1

a) What are the disadvantages of using nitrous oxide as part of a general anaesthetic for major surgery? (70%)
b) What are the benefits? (20%)

### Additional Notes
The ENIGMA Study Group has made the subject of one of the oldest agents used in anaesthesia highly topical again. As the anaesthetic community is currently firmly split on the merits and risks of nitrous oxide use, a question is likely to be along the lines of understanding both sides of the controversy

### Answer
a) The disadvantages of using nitrous oxide as part of a general anaesthetic are:
   Postoperative nausea and vomiting.★★
      Substantiated by level 1 evidence (Apfel, 2004, or ENIGMA, 2007).
   Recovery quality worse in nitrous limb in ENIGMA.
   Air space expansion★★
      Especially in pneumothorax, bowel obstruction, neurosurgery, middle ear surgery.
   Megaloblastic anaemia★
      Nitrous oxide interferes with vitamin B12 and folate metabolism by oxidising cobalt irreversibly, inactivating methionine synthetase. 1 hour exposure produces a 50% reduction in activity.
   Immunosuppression★
      Good laboratory data implicating various mechanisms.
      Neutrophil and monocyte migration is depressed by nitrous oxide.
      Methionine synthetase is required for normal bone marrow function.
      The wound infection rate was worse in the nitrous limb in ENIGMA.
   Nerve and spinal cord toxicity★
      Sub-acute combined degeneration of cord.
      Excitotoxicity. This is the spiralling process of nerve cell death following injury. This process is worsened by nitrous oxide.

Nitrous oxide produces cerebral blood flow / cerebral metabolic oxygen requirement mismatch.

Hypoxia✶

Atelectasis✶

Atelectasis and pneumonia worse in nitrous group in ENIGMA.

Adverse circulatory effects

May increase pulmonary artery pressure.

May activate sympathetic nervous system.

Homocysteine and myocardial ischaemia.

Homocysteine remains elevated for 1 week post $N_2O$.

Homocysteine is an independent risk factor for coronary artery and cerebrovascular disease.

Carcinogenicity, and occupational exposure

Industrial risks

Ozone depletion

b) The benefits of using nitrous oxide are:

Analgesic✶

Short-acting✶

Rapid onset✶

Reduced risk of awareness

Pleasant smell

Long-standing safety record

MAC sparing

Cheap

Well established, in terms of both understanding of how to use and the infrastructure in place for its use.

## References

Apfel CC, Korttila K, Abdalla M, Kerger H, Turan A, Vedder I, et al. A factorial trial of six interventions for the prevention of postoperative nausea and vomiting. *N Engl J Med* 2004; **350(24)**: 2441–51.

ENIGMA Trial Group. Avoidance of nitrous oxide for patients undergoing major surgery: a randomised controlled trial. *Anesthesiology* 2007; **107**: 221–31.

Myles PS. A review of the risks and benefits of nitrous oxide in current anaesthetic practice. *Anaesth Intensive Care* 2004; **32**: 165–72.

## Question 2

a) What are the factors that determine the amount of fluid moving through a tube per unit time (flow)? (50%)

b) Anaesthetists often refer to the size of medical tubes using the French or the Gauge system. What are these systems and how do they differ? (40%)

## Additional Notes

Everyone seems to know the Hagen-Poiseuille equation but remember it only applies to laminar fluid flow in tubes.

## Answer

a) Flow in tubes can be laminar or turbulent and the tipping point is determined by the Reynolds number.✶✶

Laminar flow

Molecular flow at the edges of the tubes is slower than the centre.✶ Flow can be determined by the Hagen-Poiseuille equation✶✶:

$$\text{Flow} = \frac{\text{Pressure gradient along tube} \times \text{tube radius}^4 \times \pi}{8 \times \text{fluid viscosity} \times \text{tube length}}$$

N.B. Viscosity is defined as the resistance a fluid offers to the motion of a solid through it. Units are in Pascal seconds (Pa·s)

Reynolds number
Describes the point at which flow changes from laminar to turbulent. For numbers below 2000 flow tends to be laminar, 2000–4000 the flow pattern is a mixture and above 4000 the flow is mainly turbulent.*

$$\text{Reynold's number} = \frac{\rho W D_0}{\eta}$$

Where $\rho$ = density of the liquid
$W$ = flow velocity of the liquid
$D_0$ = orifice diameter and
$\eta$ = viscosity

Turbulent flow
Tends to occur when the tube is unevenly shaped,* has rough walls,* when flow is through an orifice* or around sharp corners* or, as predicted by the Reynolds number, when flow velocity is too high.
The physics governing turbulent flow is complicated but roughly speaking turbulent flow is proportional to radius squared, the square root of the pressure gradient and the reciprocal of tube length and fluid density.*
For a given pressure difference you will have a lesser flow with turbulent rather than laminar flow, which explains why Heliox may be helpful in asthma treatment.

b) The term French (often abbreviated to Fr or FR) is the measurement of the outer diameter of a tube.** It is most commonly used to describe urinary catheter, endobronchial suction catheter or chest drain size.* In the French gauge system, as it is also known, the diameter in millimetres of the tube can be determined by dividing the French size by 3 (or $\pi$ to be precise); thus an increasing French size corresponds with a larger diameter catheter.**

The Stubs Iron Wire Gauge system (also known as the Birmingham Wire Gauge) is used to measure the diameter of needles,* cannulae* and suture wires.* It was originally developed in early nineteenth-century England for use in wire manufacture, and it began appearing in a medical setting in the early twentieth century.
Each gauge increment roughly correlates to multiples of 0.01 inches, but the system is not truly linear. In medical practice there is often a wide variation in the actual diameter of needles described as a certain gauge size. The needle gauge is inversely proportional to its diameter, so the larger the gauge number, the narrower the diameter** (i.e. opposite of the French system).

### Reference
Ahn W, Bahk J, Lim Y. The 'Gauge' system for medical use. *Anesth Analg* 2002; **95**: 1125.

## Question 3

a) Describe a system for classifying subarachnoid haemorrhage (SAH) severity. (30%)
b) Write a checklist for the intensive care management of a patient with SAH requiring ventilation. (60%)

### Additional Notes
This question only asks for one system in part (a). The most common systems are shown in our answer, but you should only describe one. If you spend more than 4

minutes on the first section, you will miss out on time required to score the 60% of points that lie in part (b).

## Answer

a) The two clinical scales most commonly used are the Hunt and Hess★ and the World Federation of Neurological Surgeons (WFNS)★★ grading systems. The Fischer scale classifies SAH based on CT scan appearance and quantification of subarachnoid blood.

Hunt and Hess grading system:
Grade 1   Asymptomatic or mild headache.★
Grade 2   Moderate-to-severe headache, nuchal rigidity, and no neurological deficit other than possible cranial nerve palsy.★
Grade 3   Mild alteration in mental status (confusion, lethargy), mild focal neurological deficit.★
Grade 4   Stupor and/or hemiparesis.★
Grade 5   Comatose and/or decerebrate rigidity.★

WFNS scale:
Grade 1   Glasgow Coma Score (GCS) of 15, motor deficit absent.★
Grade 2   GCS of 13–14, motor deficit absent.★
Grade 3   GCS of 13–14, motor deficit present.★
Grade 4   GCS of 7–12, motor deficit absent or present.★
Grade 5   GCS of 3–6, motor deficit absent or present.★

Fischer scale (CT scan appearance):
Group 1   No blood detected.★
Group 2   Diffuse deposition of subarachnoid blood, no clots, and no layers of blood greater than 1mm.★
Group 3   Localised clots and/or vertical layers of blood 1mm or greater in thickness.★
Group 4   Diffuse or no subarachnoid blood, but intracerebral or intraventricular clots are present.★

In all these systems, the higher the score, the worse is the prognosis.★★ The Hunt and Hess and the WFNS systems correlate well with patient outcome.★ Fischer is useful in predicting the likelihood of symptomatic cerebral vasospasm.

b) Checklist for the intensive care management of a patient with SAH:
Airway:
Tracheal intubation for GCS < 8 or rapidly decreasing GCS.★★
Avoid compression of neck veins from ties for the tracheal tube.★

Ventilation:
Maintain adequate oxygenation using a minimum of 5cm PEEP. Increase as clinically appropriate. Aim for $PaO_2$ > 13kPa.★★
Maintain $PaCO_2$ 4.0–4.5kPa.★★
Treat neurogenic pulmonary oedema with diuretics and increased PEEP.★

Circulation:
Avoid hypotension and treat with inotropes or vasopressors if necessary (norepinephrine).★★
Treat hypertension (> 160mmHg systolic) with increased sedation and/or labetalol.★★

Nursing:
Nurse 15–30° head-up angle.★★
Keep head in neutral position.
Regular neurological observations.★★

Monitoring:
  Arterial line.★★
  Central venous line★★ via femoral or subclavian veins.★
  Maintain blood pressure at 'high normal' values for patient.★★
  Give intravenous fluids – 3 l/day minimum. Monitor with CVP and/or
  transoesophageal Doppler.★

Drugs:
  Sedation with propofol ± opiate infusions .★
  Paralysis with atracurium infusion if coughing despite adequate sedation.★
  Regular nimodipine (either orally 60mg 4-hourly or 1–2mg/h
  intravenously).★★
  Treat increased blood sugar with insulin infusion.★ Aim for tight control
  of blood sugar (4.0–6.5mmol/l).

Miscellaneous:
  Urinary catheter.★
  Nasogastric tube.
  DVT prophylaxis with TEDs and intermittent calf compression.
  Avoid hyperthermia (> 37.5°C).★
  Close, regular liaison with neurosurgical team.★
  Repeat CT scan if clinically deteriorates.★

## Reference

Wilson SR, Hirsch NP, Appleby I. Management of subarachnoid hemorrhage in a non-neurosurgical centre. *Anaesthesia* 2005; **60(5)**: 470–85.

## Question 4

A patient 2 days post emergency laparotomy for duodenal perforation and four quadrant peritonitis is still ventilated on ITU due to evolving acute respiratory distress syndrome (ARDS). Having been in sinus rhythm at 100bpm she suddenly goes into atrial fibrillation (AF) at a rate of 160bpm.
  a) What are the possible causes? (30%)
  b) Outline your immediate management. (60%)

## Additional Notes

AF is the most common, sustained, cardiac arrhythmia in the critically ill and is associated with adverse outcomes. Whether this association is a reflection that 'sicker' patients are more likely to go into AF in the first place rather than AF being an independent risk factor per se is unclear. With an ageing demographic, pre-existing AF is increasing in frequency. The more unwell the patient the more likely they are to develop AF. Atrial contraction contributes 20–30% of ventricular volume, a contribution that increases with age. Thus loss of this atrial 'kick' may result in considerable haemodynamic instability in the critically ill. It is fair game for the exam and the answer has to be more than intravenous amiodarone, stat!

## Answer

a) Causes can be divided into pre-existing and acquired risk factors:
  Pre-existing:
    Age★ (the older the more likely)
    Pre-existing cardiac disease.★★ Ischaemic heart disease, cardiomyopathy, valve disease,★ or conduction abnormalities
    Hyperthyroidism★★
    Known paroxysmal AF★

Acquired:
  Hypoxia*
  Systemic inflammatory response syndrome*
  Sepsis*
  Severity of illness (i.e. the higher the APACHE score the greater the risk)
  Electrolyte abnormalities** (e.g. hypomagnesaemia, hypokalaemia)
  Drugs** (e.g. inotropes, antibiotics, antifungals)
  Hyper- and hypothermia*
  Central venous catheters (both during placement and while in situ)
  Hypovolaemia*

b) Management depends on whether the patient is haemodynamically compromised or not.**
In all situations stop any obvious triggers,** observe vital signs,** obtain a 12-lead ECG,** check a blood gas for electrolytes,** acidosis* and PaO$_2$.*
If significantly haemodynamically compromised then early cardioversion may be necessary.** Remember that this should be delivered as a synchronised shock.* An initial energy of 200J delivered biphasically is associated with a higher success rate than lower energy levels.*
If the patient is not haemodynamically compromised then look for and treat the underlying cause.** A fluid bolus may help,* as will ensuring the serum magnesium** and potassium** are in the high end of the normal range.
If the underlying cause has not been identified or has failed to respond to treatment then the decision needs to be made between rhythm and rate control.**
The vast majority of studies comparing the two strategies have been done in a non-ITU patient population, making extrapolation of the results difficult. However, to date there is no clear evidence that one is superior to the other.*

Rate control:
  In non-ITU patients digoxin** either alone or in combination with a β-blocker or calcium channel antagonist is effective but there are clearly concerns over the negative inotrope effect** of the latter two agents.
  Amiodarone is haemodynamically well tolerated and studies suggest it is just as effective at controlling ventricular rate as well as being an effective agent for pharmacological cardioversion.**

Rhythm control:
  Can be either electrical or pharmacological.*
  Post electrical cardioversion, sinus rhythm is more likely to be sustained following pre-treatment with an antiarrhythmic agent.*
  Again amiodarone is probably the safest in the critical care setting.*

Anticoagulation:
  Incidence of thromboembolism is low within the first 48 hours of onset of AF.*
  Anticoagulation will reduce the risk of thromboembolic episodes but this should be balanced against the risk of anticoagulating a critically ill patient.*

## References
Lim H, Hamaad A, Lip G. Clinical review: clinical management of atrial fibrillation—rate control versus rhythm control. *Critical Care* 2004; **8**: 271–9. Online at http://www.pubmedcentral.nih.gov/articlerender.fcgi?artid=522829 (Accessed 28 December 2008.)
Kanji S, Stewart R, Fergusson D, McIntyre L, Turgeon A, Hebert P. Treatment of new-onset atrial fibrillation in non-cardiac intensive care unit patients: a systematic review of randomised controlled trials. *Crit Care Med* 2008; **36(5)**: 1620–4.

# Question 5

A 23-year-old previously fit and well motorcyclist has an acute, traumatic and apparently incomplete cord lesion at C7 level following a road traffic accident 4 hours previously. The surgeons need to take him to theatre for cervical spine stabilisation and also repair of a comminuted compound wrist fracture.

Outline the anaesthetic problems together with possible solutions pertinent to this case. (90%)

## Additional Notes

This is a clinical case that needs some sorting out so it is potentially a good discriminator for the examiners. There are approximately 1000 new cases of spinal cord injury in the UK each year and they are often associated with other injuries so at some point you are likely to come across a case like this in your anaesthetic practice. Remember not to include autonomic dysreflexia in your answer – that comes approximately 2 weeks post-injury at the earliest. Similarly suxamethonium is safe this early (but not from approximately 72 hours to 9 months post-injury).

## Answer

Respiratory muscle involvement
> Problem: there is likely to be complete intercostal paralysis though diaphragmatic function should be preserved.★★
> Solution: postoperative ventilatory support may be needed so provision must be made for a critical care bed.★

Transfer of the patient
> Problem: the patient needs to be transferred with full spinal precautions★★ onto the operating table and then into a prone position.★★ There is an obvious risk of further cord damage.
> Solution: having lots of help★★ with transfer and positioning from an experienced team★ with clear leadership★ is essential.

Spinal shock
> Problems: all reflex activity is lost.★★ Characterised by hypotension and bradycardia due to unopposed vagal parasympathetic tone due to loss of sympathetic tone and myocardial dysfunction.★
> Patients are prone to pulmonary oedema due to loss of cardiac sympathetic stimulation affecting myocardial contractility.★
> Solutions: full monitoring is essential including an arterial line and central venous access.★★ Judicious fluid loading and use of vasopressors may be necessary.★
> Fluid preloading prior to intubation and use of atropine or glycopyrrolate to reduce bradycardic response to intubation may help.★

Securing of airway
> Problems: this may be difficult secondary to poor airway positioning due to immobilisation and the possibility of pre-vertebral swelling due to haematoma.★
> Bronchial hypersecretion can be an issue.★
> Gastric stasis is likely to be present.★
> Solutions: the need for a rapid sequence induction★★ due to gastric stasis needs to be balanced against intubation difficulty★★ so an awake fibreoptic intubation may be necessary.★
> Pretreatment with glycopyrollate may help reduce secretions.★

Venous thromboembolism
> Problem: increased risk of thromboembolism balanced against bleeding risk due to surgery.★
> Solution: pneumatic compression devices, TEDS and avoidance of hypovolaemia.★

Blood loss
Problem: there can be significant blood loss intraoperatively✶ and length of surgery may be prolonged.✶
Solution: warmed fluids and warming devices and close temperature monitoring.✶ Cell salvage devices.

Length of surgery
Solution: meticulous care of pressure points.✶

## References

Veale P, Lamb J. Anaesthesia and acute spinal cord injury. *Contin Educ Anaesth Crit Care Pain* 2002; **2(5)**: 139–43.
Allman K, Wilson I. Anaesthesia in spinal cord lesions. *Oxford handbook of anaesthesia*. Oxford University Press. 2002; 180–5.

# Question 6

a) What is the transverse abdominal plane? Describe the afferent nerve supply blocked by deposition of local anaesthetic in this plane. (30%)
b) What are the indications for anaesthetic blockade of the transverse abdominal plane? (20%)
c) How may anaesthetic blockade of the transverse abdominal plane be performed? (40%)

## Additional Notes

This block was first described in 2001. Several papers since then have indicated this to be an extremely promising technique and it is one which is catching on quickly at a national level if not at an international level. Add to this its relative simplicity and safety profile and we have a block which may appeal to the examiners as much as it appeals to clinicians.

## Answer

a) The transversus abdominis fascial (transverse abdominal) plane is located between the fascial coverings of the transversus abdominis and internal oblique muscles.✶✶ It extends from the costal margin superiorly, to the iliac crest and inguinal ligament inferiorly and the linea alba medially.✶✶
Local anaesthetic deposited in this plane exerts its effects on the ventral neural afferents of T6–L1✶ which supply the anterior and lateral abdominal wall.
These afferents course through the transverse abdominal plane, giving off a lateral cutaneous branch in the mid-axillary line before continuing anteriorly to pierce the internal and external oblique muscles and supply the skin of the anterior abdominal wall as far as the midline.✶✶
Thus anterior and lateral abdominal wall anaesthesia may be achieved by deposition of local anaesthetic in this plane.

b) Indications
Surgery involving incision of the anterior abdominal wall,✶✶ e.g. laparotomy, radical prostatectomy, open cholecystectomy, inguinal herniorrhaphy and caesarean section (under general anaesthetic).
Particularly useful when centro-axial anaesthesia is contraindicated✶ (e.g. bleeding diatheses), unwise (e.g. septic patient, spinal abnormality), difficult (obesity) or when the landmarks for abdominal field block are unclear (e.g. ilioinguinal block).

c) Patients must be fully consented and have intravenous access in situ.
The block should be performed in a clean well-lit environment with resuscitation drugs and equipment and fully trained assistance available.✶✶
A fully aseptic technique is used with the patient supine under general anaesthetic. The Triangle of Petit (see Figure 20) is identified by palpation:

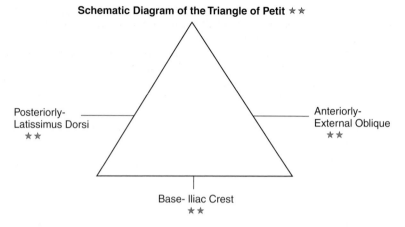

**Schematic Diagram of the Triangle of Petit** ✶✶

Posteriorly-
Latissimus Dorsi
✶✶

Anteriorly-
External Oblique
✶✶

Base- Iliac Crest
✶✶

Figure 20

A 22G 50–100mm block (blunt) needle is inserted just above the iliac crest in the coronal plane at 90° to the skin. Two 'pops' indicate passage of the needle through the fascia of external and then internal oblique, at which point the needle tip is in the transverse abdominal plane.✶✶
Levobupivacaine 0.375%✶ at a dose of up to 1mg/kg is injected incrementally after aspiration to exclude intravascular puncture. Repeated aspiration is carried out after every 5ml injected.
The same injection is carried out on the contralateral side.✶✶
Monitor carefully for signs of local anaesthetic toxicity and block efficacy following surgical incision.
The use of ultrasound may improve needle placement and therefore block efficacy.✶

### Reference
McDonnell JG, O'Donnell B, Curley G, et al. The analgesic efficacy of transversus abdominis plane block after abdominal surgery: a prospective randomised controlled trial. *Anesth Analg* 2007; **104**: 193–7.

## Question 7

A 71-year-old gentleman becomes steadily more confused during transurethral resection of the prostate gland (TURP) under spinal anaesthesia. You suspect TUR syndrome.
a) What is the mechanism for this condition? (30%)
b) What is the management? (30%)
c) How can the risk of developing this be reduced intraoperatively? (30%)

### Additional Notes
Another surprise to us that this has not been asked before as it is a discrete topic, an anaesthetic emergency and involves some basic science. Remember, there are many other causes of intraoperative confusion. This is a question that under exam conditions requires lists and bullet points, NOT an essay.

### Answer
a) The problem with the irrigation fluid used is that it needs to be non-conductive,✶ non-haemolytic✶ and must have neutral visual density.✶ Traditionally the only

solutions that could be used were electrolyte-free ones.✶ Recently, new resecting systems have come onto the market that use normal saline✶ but currently only approximately 15% of surgeons are using them.

The symptoms are caused by a combination of intravascular volume overload,✶✶ dilutional hyponatraemia✶✶ and intracellular oedema.✶✶

There may be additional problems due to glycine absorption such as visual impairment✶ and depressed conscious level,✶ glycine being an inhibitory neuro-transmitter.✶

Hypothermia can exacerbate the problem due to the large volume (up to 5 litres) of room-temperature fluid absorbed.✶

b) Like most emergency scenarios, initial management should be along the 'Airway, Breathing, Circulation' lines.✶✶

If still operating, ask the surgeon to diathermy all bleeding points and terminate surgery as soon as possible.✶

Insert an arterial line as regular blood gas analysis is likely and take baseline bloods for $Na^+$, $K^+$ and osmolarity.✶

Stop any intravenous fluids that may be being administered.✶

Call for senior help if appropriate as well as alerting the critical care team early on.✶

It may be necessary to intubate and ventilate the patient if he becomes obtunded.✶

Give furosemide 40mg intravenously and monitor response.✶

If $Na^+$ is very low (<120mmol/l) consider administration of hypertonic saline. Aim to raise the $Na^+$ by no more that 0.5mmol/l/hr.✶

c) Fluid absorption occurs in all cases at a minimum of 20ml/min so even in the most perfect of situations there remains a small (approx. 1% risk) of developing TUR syndrome.✶ There are a number of ways to minimise this risk:

Keeping the pressure of the infused solution to a minimum; i.e. don't put the bag of fluid too high above the patient.✶

Using a TURIS (transurethral resection in saline) technique. This uses a bipolar resectoscope, thus allowing normal saline for irrigation.✶

Limiting the duration of surgery to less than 1 hour. There is an exponential rise in incidence of TUR syndrome after that.✶

The more experienced the surgeon the better (faster and less bleeding).✶

Use of a regional technique so the patient's conscious level can be monitored.✶

Use of an alcometer (expired breath ethanol-level monitor) to allow early detection of irrigation fluid absorption.✶

Ensure patient has normal sodium concentration prior to surgery✶ and that heart failure is well controlled✶ as both are risk factors for TUR syndrome.

Ensure normovolaemia.✶

## References

Gravenstein D. Transurethral resection of the prostate (TURP) syndrome: A review of the pathophysiology and management. *Anesth Analg* 1997; **84**: 438–46. Online at http://www.anesthesia-analgesia.org/cgi/reprint/84/2/438.pdf (Accessed 1 January 2009.)

Hahn R. Fluid absorption in endoscopic surgery. *BJA* 2006; **96(1)**: 8–20. Online at http://bja.oxfordjournals.org/cgi/content/full/96/1/8 (Accessed 1 January 2009.)

## Question 8

Outline
a) the potential advantages (50%) and
b) the disadvantages (40%)
    of using ultrasound guidance when performing a peripheral nerve block.

## Answer

a) The potential advantages of using ultrasound (US) guidance when performing a peripheral nerve block are:

A higher success rate.★★

The direct visualisation of nerves.★★

The direct visualisation of other anatomical structures (e.g. arteries).★★

The direct visualisation of the spread of local anaesthetic, allowing needle repositioning if maldistributed and producing more complete blocks.★★

The avoidance of side effects (avoid intra-neuronal or intravascular injection).★★

The avoidance of painful muscle contractions during stimulation.★

A reduction of the dose of local anaesthetic.★

A faster sensory onset time.★

A longer duration of blocks.★

An improved quality of blocks.

The development of new improved techniques or anatomical paths for blocks.

It may be used to diagnose unrelated conditions, e.g. venous thromboembolism.

It is satisfying to perform.

b) The potential disadvantages of using US guidance when performing a peripheral nerve block are:

It requires a high degree of training/re-training.★

It ideally requires high-level ultrasonographic equipment. Basic portable Sonosite is probably inadequate. High-resolution colour and pulsed-wave Doppler imaging is desirable.★

Financial implications (hardware, training, disposables).

There is no Level 1 evidence over nerve stimulation (and probably never will be).★

Issues with service delivery and consent. If only a few members of the department can use US guidance, should they do all the blocks? If you are a not a regular user of ultrasound, should you consent an elective patient for an US or nerve stimulator guided block by you, or delay until a colleague with ultrasound skills and training is available?

## References

Hopkins PM. Ultrasound guidance as a gold standard in regional anaesthesia. *BJA* 2007; **98(3)**: 299–301.

Marhofer P. Ultrasound guidance in regional anaesthesia. *BJA* 2005; **94(1)**: 7–17.

# Question 9

a) What is the mechanism of action of volatile anaesthetic agents? (60%)

b) Why, when you reduce the flows in a circle system to 'ultra low flow' (<500ml/min), do you need to increase the percentage of delivered volatile agent in order to maintain a steady volatile concentration? (30%)

## Additional Notes

For years it was believed that the mechanism of action of anaesthetic agents was in some way related to their oil/water partition coefficient. This, in part and in retrospect, seemed to be based on the fact that a graph producing a straight line must mean something! This has now been rejected and thanks in part to a protein found in a firefly (luciferase) and two clever people called Franks and Lieb the focus switched to the interaction between anaesthetic agents and specific proteins. Recently the GABA receptor has been implicated as the main player in volatile anaesthetic agent mechanism of action. We use these agents all the time so the College is entitled to ask about how they work.

## Answer

a) Anaesthetic agents work by disrupting chemical synaptic transmission.★ This is the process whereby an electric signal in the presynaptic neurone causes transmitter release that has an effect in the postsynaptic neurone.★

Lots of different proteins,★ e.g. ion channels,★ enzymes' and second messenger systems,★ are involved in this process and experimental evidence shows that anaesthetic agents alter all of their activity.★ However, when only clinically relevant agent concentrations are considered then the family of transmitter gated ion channels★ (TGICs), of which $GABA_A$ is one,★ become the likeliest targets for the anaesthetic agents. This group also includes neuronal nicotinic acetylcholine and 5-hydroxytryptamine receptors.

The GABA receptor is a pentameric structure arranged around a central chloride pore.★ There are different sorts of GABA receptors made up of different subunits but it is the $GABA_A$ family (of which there are approximately 30 isoforms) that there is most evidence for. They sit on the postsynaptic membrane★ and when activated release chloride ions,★★ causing hyperpolarisation★★ of the cell membrane, so augmenting an inhibitory signal★★ and inhibiting an excitatory one.★★ They are also probably involved in the mechanism of action of benzodiazepines and ethanol. Anaesthetic agents have a variable effect on $GABA_A$ receptors dependent on the $GABA_A$ isoform. Staggeringly it now seems that the mechanism of action of volatile agents involves interaction with one small portion (a four amino acid residue) of the alpha subunit of the $GABA_A$ receptor. For interest propofol and etomidate interact with a beta subunit and not an alpha subunit.

It is possible that volatile agents have other mechanisms of action★ involving potassium channels and voltage-gated sodium channels as well but work on this is at an early stage.

b) Assuming a circle has no leaks and has a 5 litre capacity, to maintain a 1% concentration of a volatile agent one will need to have 50ml of volatile in the circle system at any one time.★ As the body's compartments are still taking up volatile for the vast majority of any anaesthetic, that 50ml volume decreases with each inhalation.★
At low flow the amount of carrier gas passing through a vaporiser per unit time is low★★ hence even when fully saturated the actual amount (in this case 50ml) cannot be replaced to maintain the 1% concentration.★★ Your options are to either increase the flow (which defeats the point) or increase the dialled concentration (which is what you do).★★

## Reference

Weir C. The molecular mechanisms of general anaesthesia: dissecting the $GABA_A$ receptor. *Contin Educ Anaesth Crit Care Pain* 2006; **6**: 49–53.

# Question 10

a) How are upper gastrointestinal varices formed? (30%)
b) Describe the physical and pharmacological methods used specifically in the management of an acute variceal bleed. (40%)
c) What can be done to reduce the risk of variceal bleeds in patients known to have varices? (20%)

## Additional Notes

This question emphasises the importance of reading the question and the distribution of marks carefully. The question asks for the specific pharmacological and physical methods useful in the management of variceal bleeding; be sure in the heat of the exam to answer only this question; a generic description of the management of major haemorrhage here will score few marks.

## Answer

a) Varices are formed by a pathological process occurring in the liver★★ (e.g. cirrhosis) which leads to:
1. An increase in hepatic vascular resistance.
2. An increase in portal blood flow, which exacerbates the elevation in vascular resistance.

Together these processes produce a portosystemic pressure gradient, for which the body attempts to compensate by the production of venous collateral vessels in the form of varices.★★

b) This is a medical emergency, so approach in an ABCDE fashion.
Summon the immediate assistance of an experienced endoscopist and notify an appropriate surgeon.★★
The restoration of intravascular volume is essential, but over-transfusion of fluid or blood risks exacerbation of bleeding by elevation in portal pressure and coagulopathy.★

Pharmacological

Correct coagulopathy with vitamin K (10mg IV daily for 2 days), FFP, platelets and cryoprecipitate as directed by clotting results, or empirically.★★
The administration of terlipressin (2mg, 4 hourly for 48 hours) reduces variceal pressure and therefore bleeding by reducing the portosystemic pressure gradient.★★
Somatostatin is an alternative.
Broad-spectrum antibiotics (ciprofloxacin IV 200–400mg 12 hourly) reduce the risk of infection, bleeding and mortality.★★
Metoclopramide (10mg IV) elevates lower oesophageal sphincter tone by 17mmHg and may transiently reduce variceal blood flow.
Lactulose, thiamine and multivitamins all have a role in these patients.

Physical

Urgent upper GI endoscopy is mandatory for diagnosis (patients with varices may bleed from a peptic ulcer) and therapy,★★ the options for which are:
Sclerotherapy
Band ligation
Glue (for gastric varices)
The failure of endoscopy to control haemorrhage may warrant:
Insertion of a Sengstaken Blakemore tube.★★ This consists of gastric and oesophageal balloons (oesophageal balloon inflation only used in extremis as risks oesophageal necrosis) and gastric and oesophageal aspiration ports.
Laparotomy for portocaval or mesocaval shunting, oesophageal transection or selective decompression.★★

c) Reducing the risk of bleeding can be achieved:
Pharmacologically

Propranolol (80mg PO tds) – reduces cardiac output and splanchnic arterial flow.★★
Reduces re-bleed rate but not mortality.
Physically
Regular injection sclerotherapy or band ligation.★★
Transjugular or transfemoral intrahepatic portosystemic shunt (TIPS) is a stent placed radiologically between hepatic and portal vasculature.★★ Only available in specialised centres.

## Reference
McKay R, Webster NR. Variceal bleeding. *Contin Educ Anaesth Crit Care Pain* 2007; 7: 191–4.

## Question 11

a) What are the advantages and disadvantages of pressure-control ventilation when compared to volume-control ventilation? (40%)
b) What information would lead you to believe that a patient is ready to wean from a ventilator? (50%)

### Additional Notes
The first part of this question does not demand an illustration of the classic volume vs time, pressure vs time or flow vs time graphs. However, including one or two of these graphs may show the examiner that your depth of understanding is greater than that of someone who has just twiddled some knobs on an ICU ventilator one night. Label any graph fully; all of the labels given below would be regarded as essential.(★★)
Be careful not to go overboard with undefined abbreviations in this question.
There are multiple criteria for weaning. Know one well and be prepared to recite it.

### Answer
Pressure-control ventilation (PCV) and volume-control ventilation (VCV).

a) Advantages (see Figure 21):

**Flow/Time Graphs for Pressure and Volume Control Ventilation**

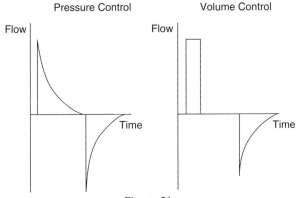

Figure 21

The square-wave rise in pressure during PCV delivers a greater volume of gas to the lungs for a given $P_{max}$ (area under flow/time graph).★★
This means that peak airway pressures are lower for a given tidal volume in PCV when compared to VCV.★★
  This minimises barotrauma (known to adversely affect outcome in ARDS) and intrathoracic pressure (which has adverse cardiovascular effects).★★
For the same peak airway pressure, the mean airway pressure will be higher in PCV.★★
  Differing gas flow patterns allow more homogeneous ventilation in PCV when compared to VCV, minimising atelectasis and maximising recruitment, especially in ARDS.★
  This results in a higher $PaO_2$.★★

PCV allows compensation for leaks – useful in uncuffed tubes (paediatrics) or during tracheostomy. VCV does not compensate for leaks.✲✲

Disadvantages
Variations in compliance or resistance will result in a variable tidal volume being delivered in PCV but not in VCV.✲✲
> This may lead to rises or falls in $PaCO_2$ and maybe $PaO_2$.✲✲
> The implication of this will depend on the patient.
> By delivering a fixed tidal volume in these situations, VCV may result in inappropriately high airway pressures which are likely to be deleterious, not seen in PCV.✲

b) This can be approached in an ABCD fashion:

> A – Protects, good cough.✲✲
> B – Muscle power:✲✲
>> −ve inspiratory pressure >25cmH_2O✲
>> compliance >25ml/cmH_2O✲
>> vital capacity >10ml/kg✲
>> minute volume <10L/min✲
>> tidal volume >5ml/kg✲
>> respiratory rate <35✲
>> index of rapid shallow breathing (resp rate/Vt) <100. Note Vt in litres.
>> – Adequate gas exchange:
>>> $FiO_2$ <0.6, $PaO_2$ >76mmHg, $PaCO_2$ <45mmHg✲✲
>>> $PaO_2/PAO_2$ >0.35✲
>>> $PaO_2/FiO_2$ >200mmHg✲
> C – No cardiac failure or critical ischaemia (temporary falls in gas exchange on weaning may jeopardise myocardial $O_2$ supply).✲✲
>> Inotropes low or reducing.
> D – Adequate pain relief.
>> Appropriate level of consciousness✲✲
>> Drugs – no neuromuscular blockers, not over-opiated.✲✲

The CROP index can be used as an objective guide but is unreliable (being effort dependent). Threshold for successful weaning = CROP 13:✲

$$CROP = Compliance \times P_{i\ max} \times \frac{(PaO_2/PAO_2)}{Resp\ Rate}$$

### References
Lumb AB. Respiratory support and artificial ventilation. In: *Nunn's applied respiratory physiology*, 4th edition. Butterworth-Heineman. 2005; 435–42.
Anaesthesia UK: Ventilation.http://www.anaesthesiauk.com/article.aspx?articleid=100421 (Accessed 29 December 2008)

## Question 12

a) How would you assess a patient's risk preoperatively of developing a venous thromboembolism (VTE)? (60%)
b) Briefly outline the non-pharmacological prophylaxis of VTE, indicating with particular reference to when each modality should be used. (40%)

### Additional Notes
This is a purely clinical question, the answer to which should pass through your mind each time you anaesthetise a patient. Be systematic and try to write down the most common answer first.

## Answer

a) The assessment of risk for VTE is based on a detailed history, examination and the results of relevant investigations.✷✷
Each of these seeks to identify the risk factors for VTE.
These can be divided into:

Patient characteristics
> Previous history of VTE✷✷
> Obesity✷✷
> Age >40✷
> Immobility, which may refer to the whole body, or be partial (e.g. one limb in plaster of paris)✷✷
> Varicose veins
> Pregnancy✷✷
> Oral contraceptive pill✷

Co-morbidities
> Malignancy✷✷
> Infection✷✷
> Heart failure (and diseases resulting in poor cardiac output)
> Trauma, particularly if this results in lower limb immobility✷✷
> Thrombophilia, e.g. lupus anticoagulant in SLE, polycythaemia

Type of surgery
> Estimated duration > 30 minutes✷
> Major pelvic or abdominal✷✷
> Major orthopaedic, e.g. hip or knee✷✷

Additional factors contributing to Virchow's Triad (venous stasis, abnormal coagulation and intimal damage)
> General anaesthesia (vs regional)✷
> Critical illness
> Dehydration✷
> Laparoscopic surgery with pneumoperitoneum

The patient's risk of VTE may then be stratified as low, medium or high based on the number of the above risk factors present.

b) Various levels of intervention.
Stop oral contraceptive pill 6 weeks preoperatively if alternative contraceptive available, accepted by the patient and suitably high-risk situation.
Early mobilisation✷✷
> Important for all patients (unless specific contraindications, e.g. patient in traction).

Graduated thromboembolic disease stockings (TEDS)✷✷
> Suitable for all surgical patients unless contraindicated by arterial insufficiency of lower limbs confirmed with ankle-brachial pressure index of <0.3.

Haemodilution✷
> Aiming for a haematocrit of 0.24–0.33 by using IV crystalloid may reduce the risk of VTE.
> Patients must, however, be able to tolerate this degree of anaemia and fluid administration (inappropriate if coronary artery insufficiency and heart failure).

Dextran 40 and 70
> Can reduce the risk of VTE.
> Adverse reactions, e.g. anaphylaxis, may, however, occur.

Intermittent pneumatic compression devices (either calf pumps or boots)✶✶
As efficacious as heparin. Useful when heparin contraindicated, e.g. heparin-induced thrombocytopenia or risk of bleeding from heparin undesirable such as in some neurosurgery.
Can be used in combination with heparin for particularly high-risk patients.

## References

Bullingham A, Strunin L. Prevention of postoperative venous thromboembolism. *BJA* 1995; **75**: 622–30.

Campbell B. Prophylaxis of venous thromboembolism. In: Allmann KG, Wilson IH, eds. *Oxford handbook of anaesthesia*. Oxford University Press. 2004; 11–14.

# Index